"For God's Sake, Don't Watch Porn for Pointers"

"For God's Sake, Don't Watch Porn for Pointers"

And 101 Other
Scraps of Wisdom from
America's Crankiest
Advice Columnist,
the Nuisance Lady

PAIGE STEIN

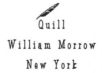

Quill
William Morrow
New York

Copyright © 1997 by Paige Stein

It is the policy of William Morrow and Company, Inc., and its imprints and affiliates, recognizing the importance of preserving what has been written, to print the books we publish on acid-free paper, and we exert our best efforts to that end.

Library of Congress Cataloging-in-Publication Data

Stein, Paige.
"For God's sake, don't watch porn for pointers" : and 101 other scraps of wisdom from America's crankiest advice columnist, the nuisance lady / Paige Stein.
p.   cm.
ISBN 0-688-15551-0
1. Conduct of life. 2. Advice columns. I. Title.
BJ1581.2.S735   1997
646.7—dc21   97-6529
CIP

Printed in the United States of America

First Edition

2   3   4   5   6   7   8   9   10

BOOK DESIGN BY JO ANNE METSCH

To Shirley and Jeremiah, Grandma and Grandpa Nuisance,
who—as they're fond of reminding me—taught me everything
I know, but not everything they know

Contents

Getting Money— Through Jobs and Other Avenues

Thank God money doesn't grow on trees. Why? Because people trying to get money are a hell of a lot funnier than people who've already got it: "Gee, let's see how can I get the most money while doing the least work or, even better, no work at all"—now that's entertainment. Hell, if they can make a Chia Pet grow overnight, why not a couple of hundred bucks? Here, buddy, here's another lottery ticket for you. Not that this is anything new for us; what was alchemy but an attempt to get gold for pretty much nothing? Thank God almost none of this hocus-pocus send-me-a-Porsche works because when was the last time you thought to yourself, "You know, there goes one hell of a nice rich guy"? Give your average guy a few million and he becomes a bigger, fatter idiot than Rush Limbaugh: "I have a six-figure salary, and you do not . . . na na na." Throw in a little fame and you end up with that modern horror of all horrors—a celebrity, "I'm on the cover of *Vanity Fair* and you are not . . . na na na."

■

He Might Be the Antichrist, but at Least He's Well Dressed

Dear Nuisance Lady,

I work for a well-known designer, a very well-known designer. You probably have several of his things hanging in your

closet. He is an absolute monster to his employees. He pays us
nothing. He regularly berates us. He'll point at someone like
they're an inanimate object and say things like, "This one wins
the stupid f——— idiot award." Yesterday, he fired one of
the secretaries because she had gained a few pounds. I dread
going to work each day because you never know if it'll be a
bad-mood day, a really bad-mood day, or a brutally bad-mood
day. I guess I should look for another job, but I've always
wanted to work in fashion and I might not get another opportunity like this. Also, won't it look bad on my résumé if I quit
for no apparent reason?

STUCK IN AN UPSCALE SWEATSHOP

Dear Stuck,

No apparent reason? You listed several appallingly apparent
reasons in your letter. The Nuisance Lady finds it funny how
everyone who works in fashion is always complaining about it—
the superficiality, the egos, the traveling, the egos, the low
wages, the egos. Yet you're always talking about the industry,
the biz, whatever. The last time the Nuisance Lady had lunch
with three of her garmento girlfriends she tried to knock herself
unconscious with a salmon steak. She couldn't take it for one
more second.

Of course you should look for another job. Get your résumé
together immediately. No doubt, everyone else in the industry
knows how horrible he is to work for. This stuff gets around.

P.S. Unless you're talking about Meyer the Buyer in Brooklyn, the Nuisance Lady definitely does not have several of his

things hanging in her closet. You obviously have no idea what people in other professions make, do you?

They Shoot Philosophers in L.A., Don't They?

Dear Nuisance Lady,

I'm in crisis. I don't know what to do. I've been offered a new job, a better job, a job with major potential for career advancement. There's only one problem, it's in L.A.—Land of the Artificial. Silicone Valley. Superficial City. Officially Designated Depth-Free Zone. Shallow Hollow. You get the idea. I love New York. I love my apartment. I love my friends. I love my doorman. I love the guy behind the counter at my corner deli. On the other hand, my family isn't here and I don't have a boyfriend or anything else that would really keep me here. I don't know. I'm so torn. Help me, Nuisance Lady. I have to give my official answer in a couple of days.

SHOULD I STAY OR SHOULD I GO?

Dear Should,

Right now there are two old Greek guys in your head. Punching each other. Parmenides, the short fat one, represents permanence, all things immutable in the universe, if you will. Heraclitus, the tall skinny one, stands for flux, constant and continual change, rolling down the river. Parmenides lands a solid right hook on Heraclitus' chin: *I'll miss my friends. I'll miss the shoestore around the corner. Where will I buy shoes in L.A.? They probably don't have shoes there.* But then Heraclitus counters with the old one-two: *It's a great opportunity. The kind I might not get again. L.A.'s not so bad. It could be fun. Good weather. Yeah, there's the weather.* In the end, one of them knocks the other one out and the fight's over. In your case the Nuisance Lady's laying odds on Heraclitus. And, don't worry, they have great shoes in L.A. The Nuisance Lady just called her friend Spacy L.A. Lacy to check—seventy-eight degrees and sunny.

P.S. From philosophy to diners—the Greeks've had an interesting progression as a people.

Isn't That Just the Sleaziest?

Dear Nuisance Lady,

My neighbor is a celebrity. He's a nice guy, and we have a friendly, say-hi-in-the-elevator, borrow-a-corkscrew kind of relationship. I happen to know, however, that he's into some pretty weird stuff, even by New York standards. I won't go into details, but suffice it to say I once had to help him bring a large person dressed in shepherdess costume to the emergency room. (It was nothing serious.)

The problem is that I've recently been having some financial difficulties. So I've been thinking about selling the story to one of the local tabloids to earn some quick cash. I really don't want to cause my neighbor any problems: ruin his life or career, etc. On the other hand, I really am one step away from, if not shopping bags on the number 6 train, then having to make some serious lifestyle adjustments—like moving out of my loft. Help me, Nuisance Lady. Be my moral compass.

NEEDY CELEBRITY NEIGHBOR

Dear Needy,

This is the kind of thing that makes the Nuisance Lady see red, yellow, and every color of the rainbow. It's what's wrong with the world as we know it. If you sell the sordid, unsightly (what could be more unsightly than a large person in a shepherdess costume?) details of your neighbor's sex life to some scandal sheet, you will be no better than the millions of moralless morons—both male and female—who have slept with celebrities and later "revealed all" for fifteen seconds of fame and some fast cash.

So, unless your well-known neighbor has done something criminal—in which case you should call the police—put down that phone and only pick it up again to call friends and family. That's what friends and family are for, to be soaked like a sheet of Bounty in moments of indigence. If you fail to fleece the kinfolk, you might even try asking, not blackmailing, your neighbor for a loan.

But My Hair Has Never Looked Better

Dear Nuisance Lady,

Can I tell you about my faithful assistant, Juarez? He's a mess. Juarez, who was formerly my hairdresser's unemployed boyfriend, needed a job. So I hired him as my assistant. I figured what better way to get in good with Rafe. He's the best I've ever had. My hair has never looked better—the cut, the color. And of course, now I never have to wait for an appointment. (Rafe is normally booked three months in advance.)

A perfect situation, right? Wrong. After nearly six months Juarez still doesn't know the slightest thing about WordPerfect. Forget PageMaker. He can't even answer the phone correctly. He always answers, "Janice Mellman's line." I haven't worked my ass off for the last eight years for a "line." It's got four walls, a desk, a door. I told him it was an office and he'd damn well better call it one.

I mean even the simplest things . . . Like a couple of weeks ago, I asked him to get me a gingerbread house for a photo layout. He comes back with a $175 gingerbread house. I said, "For God's sake, get me a stale one for ten bucks. Nobody's going to eat the damn thing." I realize this letter's pretty long, so I won't even get into vodka Fridays. I know I should fire Juarez, but I really like him. He cracks me up at least seventy-five times a day. And there's also my hair to think of. What should I do?

SOME ASSISTANCE PLEASE

Dear SAP,

Let the Nuisance Lady tell you about Lena. Lena was one of those pseudo-society-clear-out-of-the-office-at-4:45-for-a-bikini-wax type of broads. The Nuisance Lady was forced to work with her for eleven and a half long months, and let me tell you, Lena, unlike Juarez, was no laughfest. When she wasn't working on her computerized list of the "40 Richest

Men Under 40" or swapping the latest Prada bags with her second cousin Sissy, she was still doing no work. So consider yourself lucky.

Give Juarez one more shot to clean up his act. Tell him that while you don't expect him to become truly industrious or efficient (hey, you don't want to put too much pressure on the poor guy) you do require some reasonable semblance of something. Then give him a set time limit—say three months—and if he doesn't improve, start looking for another hairdresser.

Just Clowning Around

Dear Nuisance Lady,

After my husband and I spent a fortune to send our daughter to an Ivy League school, she has suddenly, after several years of sitting on the sofa, decided what to do with the rest of her life. She wants to be a clown. Not the circus kind. The kind that goes to little kids' birthdays. She's been walking around the house for weeks making balloon animals. To top it all off, she wants to borrow five hundred dollars for a course on how to be a clown, a clown-training course. I don't like to interfere in my children's lives, particularly after their twenty-first birthdays, but I really feel I have to say something here. What do you think, Nuisance Lady? Should I tell her how I feel or should I keep my mouth shut? I really find this whole thing terrifying.

BOZO'S MOTHER

Dear Bozo,

So does the Nuisance Lady. But then again, that might be because she's always had an absolute aversion to people with white faces and big red noses, whether they be Saint Patrick's Day revelers or Barnum and Bailey employees. In fact, the Nuisance Lady used to beg her mother *not* to take her to the circus.

But balloon making is better than sofa sitting. So, tell your free-loading little filly if she wants to be a clown, she has your complete support but not your five hundred bucks. If she wants to take the clown course, let her get a job and earn the tuition money herself. If it's any consolation to you, the Nuisance Lady called her friend Carol's twin sister, who is a clown (the only clown anybody knows), and she says clowning can be a financially and emotionally rewarding profession.

How Big Is His Bonus?

Dear Nuisance Lady,

As part of my Christmas bonus my boss wants to take me to the Rainbow Room for drinks and then to Tavern on the Green for dinner. He also has a blue box from Tiffany's on his desk, which he says is part of my gift. The company already gives us annual bonuses based on seniority. So this would be in addition to that, if you know what I mean. Do you think that this gift is a little bit excessive, maybe inappropriate?

ADDED BONUS

Dear Bonus,

Do the Nuisance Lady a favor. Go over to a mirror, full length. Look at your head, point to it. That is for thinking. Now, point to your little feet. Those are for dancing.

There seemed to be some confusion there. Honey, you'd have to be doing one hell of a job. And the Nuisance Lady has a feeling you ain't. Please, brokers that make their firm millions don't get that kind of treatment from the boss man. He obviously wants to see if there are little Santas on your Christmas panties. If you're serious about the corporate ladder, keep your legs crossed under the desk and suggest lunch instead. Very benign meal, lunch. Squeezed in there in between the about-to-do-it dinner and the been-done breakfast.

Those Don't Look like Nectarines

Dear Nuisance Lady,

I'm a very poor student who has a part-time job and still isn't making enough money to pay rent, buy books, and eat anything other than Kraft macaroni and cheese and frozen waffles. Recently, a friend of mine told me that she works as a model for art schools. I thought it sounded like a good way to make some much-needed money. But when I told my boyfriend about it, he hit the roof and said that he would break up with me if I even considered posing nude for strangers. Don't you think he's being unreasonable?

POSING FOR DOLLARS

Dear Posing,

Listen here, poverty-stricken little starch eater, the Nuisance Lady herself briefly toiled at that very same occupation while living in a garret in Paris, and she can assure you that in that enlightened, art-appreciating metropolis it is work well respected. The French understand that Manet's *Odalisque* or Degas's *Bathers* would hardly have been possible had a strong and patient woman not sat or stood stoically for hours on end.

Take your mate to a museum and, while there, explain to him that although you would never do anything degrading to yourself or women in general, you would be proud and happy to contribute to the creation of something of beauty. If that doesn't work, stick a bowl of fruit in front of him and tell him that to an art student there's no difference between your nude body and that tangerine.

But You Didn't Think of It, Did You?

Dear Nuisance Lady,

I'm sick of working like a little gerbil on a wheel for the small bucks. After college I got a job in a field that I was interested in and where I thought I could do some good, blah, blah, blah. But six years later I still have never been to Spain. I can't even afford to go skiing for one lousy weekend. I've had it. I want to "drink from the cup of life." I want to drain the cup dry. The only problem is that now that I've decided all I want is the big bucks, I don't know where the hell they are or how to get them. So that's my question, Nuisance Lady—where are the big bucks?

NOT EVEN SIPPING, YET

Dear Sipping,

The Nuisance Lady is not, personally, acquainted with the big bucks or even the decent-sized ones (hard to believe she doesn't get millions for doling out gems like this). But from her understanding, really big bucks come from ideas—ideas and capital. In other words, sweets, not only do you have to have one damned original, marketable idea, but then you've got to have money to get it on the market. And if you don't have your own (and who does?), that means investors. (Ones that aren't all talk and no dough are damned hard to find.)

The Nuisance Lady's aunt Esther used to live next door to the Phillipses. Mr. Phillips invented the Phillips-head screwdriver—not the screwdriver itself, just the little ridges that make a Phillips-head screwdriver different from a normal one. Everyone, particularly Uncle Harry, was always saying, "Oh, anyone could've thought of that." Well, anyone didn't—Mr. Phillips did. That's why it's the Phillips-head screwdriver and not the Harry Lefkowitz-head screwdriver.

What was your question again, honey? Oh, money. Let's see, there are still pretty nice-sized bucks to be made on Wall Street and its environs, if you're willing to sell your soul and your stomach lining. But the eighties are over and you've got to really be born to it to do that kind of thing anyway. So, just do something you love, and rewards—financial and other kinds— will come, eventually. Or not . . . but that's life.

P.S. The Nuisance Lady's annoying friend Sam is screaming

in the background, *"The Net. It's paved with gold. There's a fortune to be made on the Net."* Just passing it along to shut him up.

He's Not Exactly Robert Redford. He's a Short Japanese Man. but...

Dear Nuisance Lady,

I have one of those jobs that sound very prestigious, but really aren't all that great. (If paychecks were states, mine would be Rhode Island.) Recently, a Japanese client of ours offered me a significant amount of money to sleep with him. I said no, but now I'm reconsidering. I'm tired of working my butt off for the "company." At least in this case, I'd be working for myself and I'd get to keep all the profits. I'm not married and don't have a boyfriend right now, so I wouldn't be affecting anyone but myself. And while I don't find this man particularly attractive, he's not repulsive to me either. Plus, I have to admit the whole concept is kind of a turn-on, in a sleazy way. I know this sounds like the plot of a Demi Moore movie, but it's real life and it's a really difficult decision. Please give me some advice.

PONDERING PROPOSAL

Dear Pondering,

It is difficult to give you advice when you didn't give a dollar amount. What are we talking here, sister? Three figures? Forget it. Don't even consider anything that's not well into the fours. Some people—hell, most people—would probably get all moralistic on you and say something like *"A hooker is a hooker is a hooker."* And that's true. But who are they to judge? (It's not like giving it away for free is that great all the time either.) So, toots, it's up to you. If you can live with it—and you will have to live with it—if you think it would fulfill a fantasy, would be a crazy, kinky memory to look back on when you're in the proverbial rocking chair, go right ahead.

Old MacDonald Had a Farm and a Rolex

Dear Nuisance Lady,

I have a good job which pays very well. But it's not my dream, if you know what I mean. My dream is to be a farmer— to have a little place somewhere, maybe in Vermont—grow some corn, tomatoes, maybe even some potatoes. I know it's very difficult to make a small farm profitable, even to make a living.

I'm not scared of the hard work. I work hard now, but I also have a lot of nice stuff and a secure future to show for it. But, on the other hand, I'm a single guy and don't have anyone to think about but myself—no wife, no kids, not even a dog. Now's the time for me to live out my dream. Right?

OLD MACDONALD

Dear MacDonald,

Depends how much you like your Rolex, Farmer Brown. The Nuisance Lady's friend Ross, his dream is to be a fisher-man—not just a fisherman, but a whaler. (*Moby Dick*'s his favorite book. He's the only person who didn't skip over a few thousand pages.) He says there's a long learned tradition of whaling in his family; says they were all whalers back in the old country. But since his family were Polish Jews, you've got to wonder. Who's ever heard of whaling Jews? *"You know, Moishe, the goyim, they like whales. Me, I just take a little lox."* Then there's the fact that Poland is a completely landlocked country. So where the hell were they whaling? If they'd been Norwegian Jews, then maybe.

Anyway, call-me-Ross decided that whaling might not pay, so he stuck to Wall Street. Plus, he didn't want to be a social outcast—spat upon by whale-watchers everywhere. (Who doesn't adore those lovable fat guys of the sea?) So you have to decide if waking up to the sound of the cock crowing (the Nuisance Lady was tempted to write something here, but she won't), is more important than knowing where your next vacation is coming from. (Can't say meal because hopefully you'll at least have a meal, even if it's only a few of your own home-grown potatoes and tomatoes.)

Just remember, if you decide to go for the cash, you can still mourn the loss of your dream and get lots of melodramatic, sympathy-inducing moments out of it. Every summer Ross rents a house in Nantucket, a house with a widow's walk. There he sits, reading *Moby Dick*, tearing the pages out, and wistfully tossing them into the sea. (The neighbors don't appreciate it because the wind carries half of the pages into their backyards, but all his friends quite enjoy it. We make an annual pilgrimage every summer.)

P.S. If you go live on a farm, at least get a dog for God's sake.

Social-lite

Dear Nuisance Lady,

Since I graduated from college several years ago, I've been kind of confused. I really don't know what to do with my life. I'm from a wealthy prominent family, so I don't have to work for money. But I know I should do something . . . something to make my life meaningful. Sometimes it seems like I have too many options. It's almost overwhelming. Everyone has a path in life. How do I find mine?

MISGUIDED SOCIALITE

P.S. Please don't tell me to do charity work. I do do some, but in general I find it depressing and not at all satisfying.

Dear Misguided,

First of all, honey, people who have to work for a living don't have paths, they have jobs. But you want a path, here's one for you: Get off your lazy, self-indulgent, and no-doubt-bony ass and get a friggin' job. And not some typical socialite occupation like special-event planner, or press attaché or, even worse, contributing editor at a women's magazine.

Get a real job, something that you can throw your whole silver spoon–fed heart and soul into, like an emergency room nurse or a criminologist. It's your only hope of salvation. The alternative—life as a professional socialite—is unspeakable, and utterly incomprehensible. Personally, the Nuisance Lady would rather have "streetwalker" next to her name—at least you know what they do.

Too Many "Beas" Buzzin' Around

Dear Nuisance Lady,

I really want to open a country store—one that sells adorable little knickknacks, and fine linens, and handmade sweaters—like the one Carly Simon owns on Martha's Vineyard. I know I need to find the right location. Then I have to go to a bank and get a loan. What else do I need to do? I guess I'm just looking for some words of encouragement, Nuisance Lady.

BEA IN MY BONNET

P.S. That's what I'd call it, because my name is Beatrice—but a lot of people call me Bea.

Dear Bea,

Honey, you certainly ain't got any brains in your bonnet. All those "beas" buzzing around must've scared them away. First of all, the Nuisance Lady wants to see you go into a bank and say, "Mr. Loan Officer, would you give me thousands of dollars to open a store which sells, you know, really cool stuff . . . ?"

Furthermore, the last thing anyone needs is another little cutesy store selling overpriced cutesy stuff. The Nuisance Lady used to live next to a store called GODS. What did they sell, you ask? Why, gods, of course. Statues of gods, pictures of gods, cocktail napkins with little gods on them. Lots of people must wake up in the morning and say, "Honey, let's go buy a god today." (JUST GARGOYLES was right around the corner in case you didn't find what you were looking for in the god store.)

These little stores are either selling something other than

gods and gargoyles or they're owned by wives of wealthy, tax write-off types. (The Nuisance Lady doesn't know anything about Carly or her personal finances, but she'd lay odds that she ain't living off the profits from that store.) So don't even think about setting up shop until you're in a similar situation.

Dating and
Not Much Sex

Dating today is just like going shopping at one of those giant supermarkets that has everything—cans of Spam, spark plugs, control-top panty hose. There are too many choices. It's easy to get overwhelmed.

Look at it from a historical perspective. A couple of hundred years ago, you lived in a village a few kilometers outside of Krakow, what were your choices? Some turnips, a chicken, Farmer Wolenski's son down the road, or, if you were lucky, maybe the butcher's daughter. Your choice was made for you by virtue of birth and the size of your father's potato field.

Now there's all different kinds of milk and cows, and it's all being given away for free. No wonder we can't make up our minds. If it's not hair that's too pouffy, it's skin that's too transparent.

And when not even one infinitesimal fault can be found, what does today's slippery single mind do? It turns the very absence of imperfection into the greatest shortcoming of all: *I had to break up with him. He took me to nice restaurants and provided me with interesting conversation and great sex.*

So what do you do when there's just too much stuff on the shelves? Stop breaking open the wrappers and eating junk in the middle of the store. Start shopping at the corner market where the selection is much more limited. Or maybe one day you just stand in front of a plain old blue and white box of Kraft macaroni and cheese and decide that's what you really want. It's cheap, it's filling. Maybe a little fattening, but what the hell. Nothing's perfect.

■

Let's Play Doctor
(To Hell with the Patient)

Dear Nuisance Lady,

I know this is going to sound awful. But here goes: My great-grandfather is in the hospital. He's very ill. In fact, he's probably going to die. I feel very bad about this, but on the other hand, he's very old (ninety-three), and he's been sick for a while. The thing is, there's this really handsome resident who's taking care of him. I think I feel a vibe, but I'm not sure. Is it just too tacky to . . . you know? If not, how would I begin to approach it?

HOSPITAL HOTPANTS

Dear Hotpants,

Yeah, it's a little difficult to flirt in a dreary hospital room with a half-dead guy lying there kind of killing the mood; not to mention the yacking relatives sitting around asking ridiculous questions like "Should he take his medicine when the nurse brings it to him or save it for later?" (*Hey, Aunt Esther, it ain't Halloween candy. He doesn't take the medicine, there ain't gonna be any later.*)

Yep, Nuisance Lady's been there. When Uncle Freddo died, the little cardiac resident that took care of him was one hot tamale. Did the Nuisance Lady let a few tubes, monitors, not-so-pleasant odors stop her? Of course not. Next time you see that cute little medicine man, you just start talking to him about anything, anything but your soon-to-be late great-grandpa who you, of course, love very much, but you're doing everything you can for him and a girl can't curl up in bed with pictures of old, old dead relatives.

Ask him if he scuba dives. Every young doctor scuba dives. The old ones golf, but the young ones all scuba dive for some reason. From there you move on to the cup of coffee, glass of carrot juice in the cafeteria, and before you know it you're Mrs. Doctor Somebody.

P.S. Don't want to throw cold water on your hot little heart, but supposedly it's a myth that doctors make the best husbands. But what the hell—doctors, lawyers, Indian chiefs—it's all the same in the dark. Well, maybe it's a little different with the Indian chiefs.

I've Never... Well, Maybe Once or Twice

Dear Nuisance Lady,

I'm kind of new to the dating game and don't know too much about girls. There is this one girl that likes me, but she has so many boyfriends. I'm a very good friend of her brother, and he says she has a list of about twenty-five to thirty guys. Also, sometimes guys come up to him and say things like "How's your sister?" or "Tell her to call me."

I think the chemistry between us is so strong we would undoubtedly get married. But I don't want to be sharing her with so many guys. If they're just friends it's okay, but if they're having sex it's not. Should I put all my fears and doubts aside and open my heart to her? Or should I move on?

P.S. I don't mind if she's had sex once or twice, but that's about it.

PLEASE DON'T PRINT MY NAME

Dear Please,

My little jackrabbit, where to start? First, just because you have chemistry with someone does not "undoubtedly" mean you will get married, especially at your tender age. (If the Nuisance Lady had married everyone she had chemistry with, she'd have made more trips to Vegas than Wayne Newton.)

Second, do not believe anything this little chickadee's brother tells you about her sex life. In fact, do not even believe the chickadee herself on this score. As you will find when you get older, if you ask a woman—any woman—how many dance partners she's had, she will inevitably say three; not one, not a baker's dozen, but three. This does not, of course, mean that she's only made the acquaintance of three gentlemen in her life, it just means that she knows this is the answer that will not damage your fragile gentleman's ego.

So, in short, you are about to embark on a marvelous journey into the land of love, lust, heartache, torment, bliss, agony, and infatuation that is known as "Women." If you are stouthearted, your course, although it will not be steady, will be filled with adventure. As someone you should be studying in school (not Shakespeare, but Pope) once wrote, "Men, some to business, some to pleasure take; But ev'ry woman is at heart a rake." In other words, if you really like the girl, go for it, but there's nothing wrong with letting her know how you feel (if she wants to step out with you, it must be you and only you).

Even If You'd Been Living in a Cave...

Dear Nuisance Lady,

I'm desperate. Let me just start out by saying that. I'm very, very desperate. I haven't had a date in almost three years. Last week a friend of mine finally fixed me up on a blind date. It went pretty well, except for one thing. He told me that he likes to dress up as a male nurse. He just came out with it, out of the blue. I didn't know what to do, so I just kept eating my salad. I mean, I haven't been dating much lately, but that can't be normal. What do you think? Is it okay to go out with him again? He seemed pretty nice other than that.

JUST THAT DESPERATE

Dear Desperate,

Honey, first of all, where have you been living that you haven't gone on a date in three years? Even if you lived in a cave, some wandering shepherd would have happened by and asked you out on a date in the last three years. You have to be either extremely shy, extremely bitchy, or extremely unattractive.

I'm going to assume it's the first one because nothing in your letter indicates bitchiness and nobody is that unattractive. (If the Nuisance Lady's second cousin, scary Sammy Abramowitz, can get a date, anyone can.)

So, you shrinking little violet, get out there and start talking to men before you rot on the vine. I'm not even saying flirt with them, just talk to them. Everything else will follow naturally—dates, fabulous fun, miserable suffering. . . .

As far as Nursie Poo goes, it's a tough call. The Nuisance Lady can even get with the male-nurse thing, but you've got to wait until at least the fourth or fifth date to come out with something like that.

Never Date an Artist, Especially a Bad One

Dear Nuisance Lady,

I have one hell of a delicate situation to deal with. I'm dating this girl I really like. She's smart, funny, and extremely sexy. There's only one problem. She's an artist and, in my humble opinion, not a very good one. She does these awful little brown things. Sculptures, I guess you'd call them. Many of them are made out of sheep's intestines. She keeps asking me what I think about her work and, of course, I lie and say something like "Really remarkable." But now she wants me to help her get a show at this gallery that my friend owns. I discreetly approached my friend about this and he said, and I quote, "Not if Picasso himself came back to life, begged me, and offered to throw in a few freebies in the bargain." So, now I'm really in a pickle. My girlfriend keeps pressuring me, but I don't want to hurt her feelings by telling her what my friend said.

ANGUISHED OVER UGLY ART

■   ■   ■

Dear Anguished,

Yours is an extremely prosaic predicament, especially in this mecca of the arts—the good, the bad, and the downright execrable. If the Nuisance Lady had a ten-spot for every odious one-act play, fearsome piece of performance art, and egregious gallery opening she's had to attend she'd be richer than old Sammy Wal-Mart. In fact, the Nuisance Lady has just ended a year-long liaison with a guy who's unquestionably the worst actor in America.

In a sensitive situation such as this, you would be wise to continue the course of diplomacy you've already been following. The next time she pressures you, just smile sweetly and say something like, "Even though my friend really loves your work, he's not sure if his gallery is the best venue for showcasing it."

P.S. You think you've got problems. At least you didn't have to sit through a four-and-a-half-hour version of *Waiting for Godot*. No wonder Godot never showed up. The Nuisance Lady wished she hadn't.

Ode to His Coy Mistress, or Mister

Dear Nuisance Lady,

This is kind of a complicated, twisted story, but please try to follow me.

My boyfriend's sister is married to this guy who has a brother. This brother seems to pay an awful lot of attention to my boyfriend. He's always inviting him (not us) to his beach house for the weekend. He buys him expensive gifts: Italian silk ties, cashmere sweaters, etc. He's even flown him to Europe several times "just to hang out."

Then the other day I checked my boyfriend's voice mail and there were several long, long messages from you-know-who. When I told my boyfriend that I thought it was strange to leave such long messages that didn't really say anything, we had a big fight. He said I was crazy, paranoid, and disgusting for even implying what he thought I was implying. He said they were all one family now, and that you-know-who was just a very family-minded guy. What do you think? And if you're thinking what I'm thinking, what should I do? I love my boyfriend a lot but this is just too . . . you know.

SUSPICIOUS

P.S. Did I mention the fact that you-know-who never seems to be with a woman even though he's divorced, loaded, and not bad-looking for an older guy?

Dear Suspicious,

Yes, I do know and so does your boyfriend. Please—expensive sweaters, trips to Europe, long phone messages. Most mistresses would kill to be treated that well. (Not that the Nuisance Lady actually knows any mistresses.)

Intimacy between two men other than the backslapping, beer-drinking, he's-my-good-buddy-I-love-that-guy variety should always be looked on with suspicion. Take the Nuisance Lady's good friend Connie as an example. Connie's boyfriend was in some twelve-step program. He was always in some twelve-step program. Anyway, he used to have these long, long 2:00-in-the-morning phone conversations with his twelve-step partner, Bill. *"Not normal,"* the Nuisance Lady said to Connie. *"Don't be ridiculous,"* Connie replied. Two months later Connie's boyfriend was twelve-stepping out the door and into Bill's waterfront condo.

Back to you, poor dear. You must immediately take the bull by the horn, so to speak. You must confront your boyfriend and explain to him that the situation is uncomfortable. Then give him an ultimatum: you or the trips to Europe, the Armani suits, and the long weekends at the beach. If he's a real man's man, we know which he'll choose.

The Basics of Blind Dating

Dear Nuisance Lady,

What do you think of blind dates? I know this isn't the most original question, but at the moment it's very pertinent because my matchmaking friend Madge is trying to fix me up with a guy she swears is the greatest thing since guilt-free potato chips. On the one hand, I'm hesitant, especially since the last guy Madge set me up with talked about his stomach abscess for forty-five minutes and then had the unfathomable density to ask why I wasn't eating my tuna maki. But on the other hand, if I spend another night watching *Honeymooners* reruns, I'll throw myself into the Cuisinart.

BAD BLIND DATER IN BROOKLYN

Dear Bad,

Blind dating is like going into a Gap. Sometimes you find something cool and comfortable that you can keep for life and other times it's just a big waste of time. Take the case of the Nuisance Lady's last blind date, ever. It was with a pharmacist named Fredan, who smelled of frankincense and myrrh, over-whelmingly so. She and Fredan, who was five feet tall, went on a dinner cruise, a really long one. Aboard, she and Fredan feasted at a bountiful buffet where cream sauces ruled the day and then listened to a sequined song guy enthusiastically offer his rendition of *"The rhythm is going to get you. The rhythm is going to get you. . . ."* (Not kidding.)

But there is also Grandma and Grandpa Nuisance, who met on a blind date (she picked him up in her tangerine convertible with the Harris-tweed seat covers), and who will be celebrating their fifty-third could-you-believe-it wedding anniversary next week.

Settling Down to So-so Sex

Dear Nuisance Lady,

Do you think it's better to have a relationship based on deep friendship and like-mindedness, which would inevitably result in a long and satisfying life of companionship, mutual respect, and shared interests, or a life marred by loneliness, temporary gratifications, and devastating disappointments? You see, several years ago my best friend, Harry, and I made a pact that if neither of us had found true love or some rea-sonable semblance of it by the time we were fifty, we'd get married (to each other) and move to Marblehead, Massachu-setts. In the last couple of years both of us have suffered through numerous bad dates, relationships, sexual encounters, etc. Not to mention that between the two of us we've racked up three sexually transmitted diseases (disgusting, but minor ones, thank God), five broken hearts, and lost two rent-controlled apartments.

Anyway, the other day it hit me: Why put ourselves through all these years of torment? Why not just get married now and have nice lives? However, when I ran this idea past Harry, he said that we were too young to give up on the idea of true love. I say we're almost thirty, and this one great love thing is all a bunch of bull anyway, so what the hell? What do you say?

TIRED OF THE CHASE

Dear Tired,

Relax. What you're experiencing is very common. It's called the *Oh-my-God-I'm-thirty (or thereabouts)-and-I-still-haven't-found-him (or her)* panic. Under the insidious influence of this hysteria our natural instinct is to find a friend, batten down the hatches, and settle, settle, settle. But unfortunately you will find, as the Nuisance Lady and her very dear friend Milton did, that Scotch, so-so sex, and CNN do not take the place of pounding hearts, racing pulses, sweating knees, and hours of ardor. Harry is right. Don't even think of settling before sixty-five.

P.S. If, by any chance, your sudden "realization" was sparked by a secret crush on Harry, tell him, tell him immediately. Or just grab him and kiss him. After all, as the Nuisance Lady's best friend, Francie, says, *"Anything that won't kill, won't kill you."* And rejection won't kill you.

Is This Fruit Forbidden?

Dear Nuisance Lady,

I'm a recently divorced man with a grown daughter. My daughter and I have a very good relationship, and she frequently comes to spend weekends with me at the beach. She sometimes brings her friend Kyla with her. Kyla is a very, very beautiful young woman and, to be honest, I'm quite attracted to her. Do you think, under the circumstances, it would be wrong of me to ask Kyla out? I don't want to do anything to hurt my daughter or my relationship with her. However, we're all adults and I don't see why we can't handle the situation as such.

TEMPTED

Dear Tempted,

Riddle: *What's more pathetic than a recently divorced middle-aged man?*

Answer: Nothing. Absolutely nothing. Not even all the guests on all the Ricki Lake and Sally Jesse shows combined. Not even Ethics 101 taught by Professor D'Amato. Not even the Nuisance Lady's cousin Stevie's Bar Mitzvah at Great Adventure. Elderly Jewish people at a theme park. Not a good idea. Who would've thought?

Anyway, back to you, Mr. Adult. If you had any brains (in your head) you would know that no child, of any age, wants to think of their parents engaging in any activity that could vaguely be construed as sexual. Even opening up a package of Ballpark Franks with your teeth is too much. And the idea of one of your parents engaging in such activity with one of your friends is so abhorrent that just typing it on the computer screen is making the Nuisance Lady's flesh crawl. So don't risk ruining your relationship with your daughter just because you're getting a hot potato watching some young chickadee splash around in her bikini. Go out and find yourself somebody's daughter who's a total stranger to yours.

P.S. What of the splendors of dating a woman your own age? You middle-aged guys are all alike.

Sex and Death: A Not-so-Subtle Connection

Dear Nuisance Lady,

I've finally met a guy I want to have sex with and, might I say, not one second too soon. It's been eighteen long months since I broke up with my boyfriend and since then, nothing . . . until this guy. The only problem is that he seems to be encountering a run of bad luck: A week after we met, his father died. Then right after that he lost his job—on his birthday. I want to say to him, "Don't worry. There's light at the end of the tunnel. I'll have sex with you." But I guess that wouldn't be appropriate, huh? Also, even if I ever do manage to hook up with this guy, now I'm starting to worry that he's got a bad vibe. Maybe I should just steer clear of him. But then again he's so cute. What do you think?

SEXUALLY STARVED

Dear Starved,

Silly girl, words are for kids. There's no reason to "say" anything to him. Just simply (and subtly) offer him the comfort that only your soft, warm bosom can provide in this, his time of need. You will be amply rewarded by untold depths of gratitude and cute masculine vulnerability—riches that would in a ''normal'' situation take you months to mine. And don't worry about his bad vibe. The Nuisance Lady's cousin Ronald met his wife, Wanda, the same week that she was diagnosed with Lyme disease and her apartment burned down, killing her beloved cat, Winks, and forcing herself and her three impoverished roommates out into the street. And they've been happily married for seven years.

P.S. Did anyone ever tell you that you are one twisted chick? But that's okay, the Nuisance Lady likes twisted.

Hey, Be Careful; You Could Hurt Someone with That Fling

Dear Nuisance Lady,

I have worked with a client for the last year. We have enjoyed a warm working relationship and I fell victim to a major crush. I thought something might develop in the future. My plans were shattered when I found out that he's getting married in a week! What gives? You know someone for a year and they don't let on that they're engaged? A woman would never let it be unknown that she had a sweetie in her life. Don't you find this odd? What's wrong with men?

CLUELESS

■   ■   ■

Dear Clueless,

The Nuisance Lady always wonders how broads get to be as old as you—old enough to have clients—and know as little as you know. This is the typical male just-let-me-flirt-and-flatter-my-ego-a-little-before-I-walk-down-the-aisle-in-fancy-dress thing. It's very common. Women do it too, although not as often because they're too busy flashing their big rocks in your face. The Nuisance Lady was almost knocked unconscious the other day by some broad waving around her antique, emerald-cut, ten-carat, sapphire-encircled, platinum-set, diamonded-ring finger. Anyway, although your client showed very, very bad form (after all, a quick flirt here and there is one thing, but to let it go on for a whole year quite another), there is not much to be done. It does, as they say, happen. Next time though, follow this simple rule: If something concrete, like a kiss, has not occurred within six weeks, take it as a sign to move on down the line.

Don't Put Out the Fire

Dear Nuisance Lady,

I've recently started dating a man who is kind, considerate, etc. But there's one problem—his profession or, rather, our professions. He's a fireman and I'm an assistant professor of French literature. Last night I brought him to a faculty party, and it was not a flaming success. (If you'll pardon the pun.) The only thing anyone said to him all night was "Oh, so, you're a fireman." It made me very uncomfortable, as did the snickering comments from the other women present about his presumed "strength" and "stamina." They assumed that was the only reason I was dating him, which isn't the case. (Although I must admit I find the image of him walking out of a burning building with sweat pouring off his smoke-stained face incredibly arousing.) Should I try to find someone I have more in common with?

FANNING THE FLAMES

Dear Fanny,

Listen, Miss Snottypants, the Nuisance Lady's had just about enough of you—and she's never even met you. First of all, do not toss around words like "kind" and "considerate" so casually. These are not et-cetera adjectives.

As far as your Montaigne, Balzac, and Flaubert-loving friends go—and the Nuisance Lady loves Montaigne, Balzac, and Flaubert as much as the next guy—they are obviously jealous. They wish they had their own *pompiers* to warm the cockles of their envy-encrusted little hearts. (By the way, the Nuisance Lady just learned what a cockle was last weekend. It's a very, very small clam.)

Finally, a well-muscled man who goes into a burning building to save another human life for under a six-figure salary is sexy. So, get over yourself and into something French and frilly, and go pay him a surprise visit at the firehouse.

Dating—It's the Pits

Dear Nuisance Lady,

The other night at a party I was introduced to a very pretty woman. We were having a really good conversation, and I was just about to slip in the old "let me get your number," when she raised her arm to gesture and I noticed that she had very, very hairy armpits. I was surprised, shocked even, and I just couldn't get past it. I stared at her underarms the rest of the conversation and didn't ask for her number. The next day I told my best friend, and she said I was incredibly shallow and superficial. Do you agree?

HERSUTE

Dear Hersute,

The Nuisance Lady recently had a similar experience (when hasn't she?). She was at an elegant soirée having a very engaging conversation with this chap about the difference between hogs and pork bellies when her nosy friend Nan leaned over and whispered, *"He's impotent."* The Nuisance Lady wasn't even interested in this fellow, but it was incredibly disconcerting. She kept picturing him in tights and a cape with a giant yellow **I** on his chest: *Look. Over there. It's a bird. It's a plane. It's IMPOTENT MAN. Not able to leap anything.*

Anyway, it might have been a little *extérieur,* as the French would say, to get all tangled up in her armpit hair. But what the hell, we are all superficial when it comes to the aesthetics of a potential bedmate. We all have things we can't get past, so-called *deal breakers.* For the Nuisance Lady, it's noses. She can't stand men with little, turned-up, girly noses. (Imposing

Roman noses, on the other hand, drive her to distraction.) For you, it's an excess of body hair. Forget about it and find a girl who shaves.

Just Keep Those Legs Crossed, Girls

Dear Nuisance Lady,

I've never had sex. I don't know how it happened. But . . . it did. In high school I almost "went all the way," but it never felt quite right. Then, in college I went out with this devout Catholic guy who didn't believe in premarital sex. Since college the only man I've dated seriously had a "problem." (I'm not kidding.) I'm getting a little tired of waiting for true love, and am considering just having sex with someone. The problem is that now I'm embarrassed about my virginity. Should I tell the guy I'm a virgin? If so, how do I explain it?

VESTAL VIRGIN ON STATEN ISLAND

Dear Vestal Virgin,

Fascinating. The Nuisance Lady has always wondered about people who manage to stay virgins well into their twenties and thirties. You'd think it—sex—would've come up, just in the ordinary course of things.

Anyway, the Nuisance Lady obviously cannot make this decision for you. But if you decide to press on, don't, for God's sake, allow Bobo the Garbage Boy to deflower you. At least choose someone that you have deep respect and affection for—a close friend, perhaps. As to any embarrassment you might feel, don't give it a second thought. Sex, as you will eventually find out, is often embarrassing—even for the well initiated. Definitely let the guy know you're a virgin, though. Explain it exactly as you did in your letter.

If you do decide to wait for the "one," remember what Nana Nuisance always says: *"Don't save it for so long that nobody wants it anymore. Did you hear me, girls?"* Quite a contrast to what Grandma Nuisance always says: *"Just keep those legs crossed. Did you hear me, girls? Just keep those legs crossed."*

For God's Sake, Don't Watch Porn for Pointers

Dear Nuisance Lady,

I think I have a really embarrassing problem. I think I might not be able to "satisfy" a lady. I'm not 100 percent sure, but the woman I was dating broke up with me soon after we made love for the first time. (Ditto with the girlfriend before that.) I asked her if she was "satisfied" and she said yes, but maybe she was lying to protect my feelings. How can I find out the truth? I'm too embarrassed to discuss this with any of my friends.

CONFIDENCE PROBLEM

Dear Confidence,

You know what they say, *"If you have to ask . . ."* Actually the Nuisance Lady isn't sure what they say, but it ain't good. One can only hope you're not running around inanely chirping,

"Was it good for you? Was it good for you?" That's enough to make any woman leap into her Levi's and run screaming into the street, even if it's her apartment.

The Nuisance Lady suspects that your confidence problem, as you put it, is making you hesitant. (Also, the fact that you used the term "making love" is not a good sign. No self-respecting straight guy says "make love" unless he's forced to by some broad.) Women do not like hesitant men. Most women, contrary to that seventies Alan Alda myth-thing, do not even like sensitive men. They might marry them. They might bring them as their dates to weddings, but they do not like them. They like a certain devilish charm, a certain cockiness (not arrogance; there's a difference).

Anyway, the Nuisance Lady could give you a detailed description of what women like in bed and out, but she doesn't have the space. So, get some books, talk to female friends—a few beers, shots of Wild Turkey will help you get over the embarrassment. And, most important, be a little bolder—experiment, bust out. What's the worst that could happen, you'll get a few "stop thats"?

P.S. For God's sake don't watch porn for pointers. Those women are getting paid to look like they're enjoying it.

A Rose Is a Rose

Dear Nuisance Lady,

I'm deeply, madly, truly obsessed with Charlie Rose, the talk-show host on PBS. I think he's fabulous. Just the thought of him makes me giddy. I know this sounds silly coming from a grown woman (I haven't felt this way since I was in "love" with Ringo Starr). Do you know anything about Mr. Rose? Is he married? How can I meet him? How can I stop thinking about him?

A ROSE IN THE DEEPS OF MY HEART

Dear Roseheart,

I think you and Charlie might have a lot in common. Charlie seems like he too is deeply, madly, truly in love with himself. He is admittedly a good-looking, well-informed guy, but he talks over his guests. It's enough to make you wonder why he even has guests. He could just sit there with the black background and talk about whatever the hell he wants for an hour. The man even talked over Elie Wiesel for God's sake.

By the way, the Nuisance Lady's cousin Nanette, who's from Short Hills but thinks she's French, is deeply, truly, madly obsessed with Mr. Wiesel. Once she thought she saw him sipping Pernod in a Parisian bistro. Armed with copies of *The Night Trilogy,* she made the Nuisance Lady return to the same bistro for five Sundays in a row. Nanette's "Wiesel" turned out to be a Swiss pharmaceutical salesman, which was music to the Nuisance Lady's ears, as she had been extremely reluctant to involve so illustrious a personage as Wiesel in something reminiscent of an *I Love Lucy* episode.

Now, as to your questions about Mr. Rose (by the way, you've got to be a middle-aged WASPy broad; you middle-aged WASPy broads love him), the Nuisance Lady cannot waste her somewhat valuable time finding out stuff about celebrities' personal lives. What do you think this is, *Parade* magazine? But she will say, as she has countless times before, meeting celebrities in person is like New Year's Eve, Shakespeare in the Park, certain sexual positions, money-back guarantees—DISAPPOINTING.

> *P.S.* The heavy steps of the plowman, splashing the wintry mold
>
> Are wronging your image that blossoms a rose in the deeps of my heart.
>
> —WILLIAM BUTLER YEATS
>
> "The Lover Tells of the Rose in His Heart"

Is the Nuisance Lady good or what?

Where There's a Whip There's a Play

Dear Nuisance Lady,

I've just discovered something very important about myself. I'm not turned on by sex in the conventional sense. I need other stimulation—like spanking and clamping. Do you think this will involve a complete change of lifestyle? Does it make me some sort of freak?

UNCONVENTIONAL

Dear Unconventional,

Hey, buddy, what do you think this is—some perverted little sex column? Besides the Nuisance Lady has never understood the whole S&M thing anyway: too much complicated clothing, too many complicated gadgets. Who can be bothered with all the buckles, and the belts, and the zippers, and the thigh-highs, and the lace-ups, and the on/off switches?

But she did go to one of those clubs once with her second cousin, Slap-Me-Harder Sadie, arrived just in time for the show, were given front-row seats—on the nasty side of the rope. Of course, Sadie disappeared after two minutes and left the Nuisance Lady sitting there with another cousin, Joe, whose communion name she chose. (Little tip for you: Don't go to these places with family.)

The "show" turned out to be a short, stocky guy in a leather toga taking a couple of swats at a pasty, cellulite-riddled chick's ass. It would be hard to imagine two people you'd less rather see engage in sexual activity. But, if you enjoy it . . .

Drinks with Little Cherries, Never a Good Idea

Dear Nuisance Lady,

Last night I did something I never thought I'd do. Ever. I slept with a man. (I am a man. That's what makes it so bad.)

I was on vacation and I met this guy and we started talking. We drank many, many, many drinks with cherries. The next thing I know, the guy's back at my hotel room and he's kissing me on the lips. And I'm kissing him back. I can't believe it. I'm in shock. How could this have happened? It must have been all those drinks, right?

KISS ME NOT

■   ■   ■

Dear Kiss,

The Nuisance Lady's been drunk with lots of broads, but she never ended up in bed with any of them. Sorry, buddy, can't blame it on the booze. (Unless the guy slipped you a Mickey, but—don't get too excited—doesn't sound like he did.)

You, sir, are a gay man. Or at least a bisexual man. If you follow the typical path—the one all the Nuisance Lady's gay friends have—you will begin by declaring that you are a BI-sexual. And within a year, you'll be living with a stylist named Kenneth and two shih tzus.

Trying to hold that closet door shut when those hinges are squeaking like crazy, about to burst at any moment, is no fun at all. Much better to fling open the door and leap right out. Even if the door swings back and hits you in the head a couple of times, it's still better than staying in that closet—too claustrophobic.

Oh, and unless you're in a British boarding school or a Southern military academy, don't try to pass it off as only experimentation. And if you are, you're too young to be drinking all those drinks with cherries.

P.S. Just remember, there's nothing wrong with sleeping with a man, if that's who you want to be sleeping with. Having sex with a broad and imagining she's Jean-Claude Van Damme—that's bad.

Family—The Root of All Insanity

Even though your first instinct is to deny that you are one of these people, you have to fight it. You want to believe that the mother ship accidentally left you—or them—behind. You want to believe that your real parents, your birth parents, are living in Indiana someplace, but you mustn't let yourself. You have to embrace them as your own, because— believe it or not—they are. There's no escaping it. If you try and break away from the pack, they'll tear you to shreds with their fangs of guilt and their tales of winter-long labor pains. No, there's nothing to do but climb to the highest split-level ranch-house rooftop and cry out, "These people are crazy and I am one of them. I'm crazy too. And in twenty or thirty years I'll be just like one of the old ones. And, after that, I'll be just like one of the dead ones the old ones are always talking about. This is my fate and I've accepted every excruciating moment of it."

What Happened to Packin' Lunch Boxes?

Dear Nuisance Lady,

My problem is my mother, or rather, my mother and her gun. After one of her neighbors was robbed she decided to purchase a handgun for self-protection. I'm ordinarily an advocate of gun control, but when it comes to my mother, I am

a fanatic. I don't mean to be unkind, but my mother has the hand-eye coordination of a one-eyed cat who's just had his whiskers clipped off. Baby bats have better eyesight. My brother and I have tried everything to convince her not to get a gun: We offered to install a high-tech alarm system, cited statistics on the number of people killed by their own guns. Nothing has worked. Do you have any suggestions, Nuisance Lady? I'm weak-kneed with worry.

DESPERATE DAUGHTER

Dear DD,

Listen, little comrade in arms, you think you've got problems. The Nuisance Lady's own mother, much to the dismay of many, keeps a .57 Magnum in her underwear drawer. Despite the oh-so-earnest entreaties of the Nuisance Lady, assorted family members, and numerous neighbors, she has stubbornly, like a Mississippi mule on a summer Sunday, refused to rid herself of the rod. So far, her only targets have been a few pesky snapping turtles who live (or lived) in the pond in her backyard. (She has also repeatedly ignored the "rantings" of the sheriff's department, which has politely informed her that it's illegal to shoot off your six-gun in suburbia.) So, sister in sorrow, the only thing the Nuisance Lady can say is: *"Don't give up the fight."* You might also want to make a contribution to the gun-control lobby. The Nuisance Lady's check is already in the mail.

P.S. The one group that's not boycotting Mama Nuisance is the Society for the Protection of Rare Birds—Certainly Not Turkeys—That Don't Fly. It seems the snapping turtles had been killing the no-flying birds, cutting them off at the knees. They keep giving her plaques, little ceramic statues of wingless birds. Like she didn't have enough useless tchotchkes all over the house.

You Don't Have to Be Born Jewish to Make a Mean Blintz

Dear Nuisance Lady,

I'm a Jewish girl who's trapped in an Episcopalian's body. As long as I can remember I've had this longing—you could say, calling—to be one of the chosen people. I make perfect potato latkes, can sing all the songs from *Fiddler on the Roof,* and am saving money for a trip to Tel Aviv.

I'd really like to come out of the "closet," or from under the chuppah, but I'm terrified of the threats of disownment, disinheritance, and disembowelment, which would inevitably flow from my devout family. On the other hand, I don't know how much longer I can continue living with this theistic torment.

BETH ISRAEL

Dear Beth,

As quirky as your quandary is, it's not novel to the Nuisance Lady. Her ambiguous friend Arthur is also a Jewish woman trapped in the body of a Christian. And he's also got that gender thing working against him.

He, too, bakes blintzes you would barter your best friend for, is El Al's favorite frequent flier, and has been known to belt out *"Match maker, match maker, make me a match . . ."* after a couple of beers. Perhaps the two of you could start a support group, if one doesn't already exist.

Also, you might want to meet with a rabbi on the sly. Discuss all this with him.

P.S. Did you know the Nuisance Lady's really a druid?

You Might Want to Spring for the Full Body Wax

Dear Nuisance Lady,

My husband and I recently went to visit my daughter and son-in-law in Rio. I couldn't help noticing the amount of weight that my daughter had put on. I was very surprised when we went to the beach and she disrobed to reveal a thong bikini, or *tanga* as they're called in Brazil. We've made plans to go on a holiday cruise and I would really prefer that my daughter not wear her *tanga*. My husband, however, says I shouldn't say anything to her because everyone wears them in Brazil and my daughter, and son-in-law, are obviously satisfied with her body. What do you think?

NERVOUS NELLIE

Dear Nellie,

Personally, the Nuisance Lady wouldn't wear a *tanga* even if she had the butt of a thousand-and-one Levi ads. But that's beside the point. Either your daughter is, as you say, satisfied with her body—which in this day of liposuction and super-models is extremely rare—and her strength of character should be applauded. Or she feels very self-conscious about her weight gain and doesn't need you opening your big mother-mouth saying stuff like *"It wouldn't hurt you to lose a few pounds."*

You want to be like the Nuisance Lady's aunt Attritia, who was always hounding the hell out of her daughters, watching every ounce, every morsel? One of them is now a three-hundred pound-gender-bending lumberjack who lives upstate with a parolee and lots of snakes, and the other one lives in a big house on Long Island and hasn't eaten solid food since '79. Your sensible spouse is completely correct—keep your mouth shut and let your daughter *tanga* the day away. You could even join her.

From Russia Without Love

Dear Nuisance Lady,

My daughter brought her new boyfriend over for dinner the other night and my husband and I almost died. He's from some republic in the former Soviet Union—Turgenev, Cheznev, or something like that. He's got a beard—a beard like Abraham's, a beard from the Old Testament. He's got no teeth, or not many anyway. And he makes noises—strange noises. All during dinner, he's making these noises. We couldn't even eat the pot roast, the noises were so loud.

The worst part is, she met him in a cab. He was driving the cab and she was riding in it. Can you believe that? We did not raise our daughter to pick up taxi drivers. What's next, the handyman? What should we do about this? We're considering telling her that unless she stops seeing this man we're going to cut off the little something "extra" that we send her every month.

RILED OVER RUSSKIE

Dear Riled,

If you think Ivan the Cabbie is bad, you should see some of the guys the Nuisance Lady and her sisters have brought home: Like Jeb—a boyfriend of the Nuisance Lady's much-older-sister Maxie—who wore purple eyeliner, stocked cans in his basement in case of nuclear disaster, and never, to the best of anyone's knowledge, spoke a word. Maxie did all his talking for him: *"Jeb says he has to leave now." "Jeb says he likes lasagna."* It was amazing. No one could figure out how they did it. You couldn't see lips moving or anything.

Anyway, your daughter will go through a lot of losers before she picks the loser she's going to marry. Just have patience and perseverance and a sense of the absurd, and you will survive. Also, if you want to cut off the "extra," do it—but not because of who she's dating.

Didn't You Mess Around with My Little Sister?

Dear Nuisance Lady,

I'm writing to you about my sister, who is a big tramp. Guys are always calling the house and she goes out on lots of dates with lots of different guys. She doesn't seem to be serious about any of them. I don't have any proof that she's sleeping with these guys, but I don't think it's any way for a girl to act. Do you?

P.S. I've tried talking to her about it, but she says she's over eighteen and can do what she wants.

SCANDALIZED BY MY SLUTTY LITTLE SISTER

Dear Scandalized,

You think your sister is a bit on the wild side? You should've seen the Nuisance Lady's much-older-sister Maxie in her anything-goes, pre-AIDS, Danskin-wearing, disco days. What a ho'doggy! Now as for you, little Missy, the tone of your letter sounds a little too sanctimonious. Are you sure there isn't just a touch of sibling rivalry, perhaps even jealousy, tainting your concern for your sister? As your sister says, she is old enough to make her own decisions, sexual and otherwise.

You could leave an economy-size box of condoms on her bed just to show you care. That's what Maxie is planning to do for her daughters, who show early signs of following in their mother's footsteps. As of late they've taken to asking the little boys in their Gymboree class if they want to see their chi-chis. Then, without waiting for a response, they pull their little flowered sundresses up sky-high. As Nana Nuisance always says, *"When it comes to kids, you get what you deserve."*

He's No Poet and
He Doesn't Even Know It

Dear Nuisance Lady,

How do you tell someone that they have absolutely no talent? My nephew, bless his heart, wants to be a poet. But, to be frank, he's read me a lot of his poetry and it's god awful. One of his recent poems began, *"Sitting on a city bench glaring at big red pumpkins."* I don't want to hurt his feelings because he's such a sweet boy, but on the other hand, I don't want him to waste his life doing something he's not cut out for.

VERY UNPOETIC

Dear Very,

The Nuisance Lady was going to say that talent is a subjective thing; one man's genius is another man's "sucks." But after reading that pumpkins thing she has to agree—the kid ain't no poet. Why is he glaring at the pumpkins? Is he mad at them? Did they do something? And why are the pumpkins red? Why aren't they orange like every other pumpkin in the world?

Anyway, how is your nephew planning to make a living? Even Auden couldn't make money in this environment. He obviously has to have another job. (Unless he's independently wealthy, in which case, who cares? Let him run around reciting bad poetry to the butler all day.)

As long as your nephew's limericks don't keep him from working, don't worry about it. Just let him read you a poem once in a while and if he tries to go on (poets, particularly bad ones, are like the Energizer bunny—they just keep going and going), smile and say, "You know, I'd really like to savor that awhile."

P.S. If he needs a job, maybe he can work down at the garage with the Nuisance Lady's cousin Mike. He's a philosopher.

Oh, You're Going All Right...

Dear Nuisance Lady,

If I spend one more Christmas in a retirement community in Arizona, I'm going to kill somebody—most likely my parents. Every year they buy me a ticket to go visit them at Sunnydale Village. And every year I'm dying to say no, but every year I go. It's sucking the life right out of me. A hot, dry Christmas watching retired FBI guys (Dad is a retired FBI guy) play golf is not my idea of a splendid holiday. Of course, every year I try to get out of it, you know, hint around. But every year my mother says, "Oh, well, if you don't want to come . . ." (We all know what that means, don't we?) But this year I'm going to make a stand. Even though my bags are packed and my ticket came in the mail three days ago, I'm not going. Maybe. Is that too horrible?

NOT ARIZONA AGAIN

Dear Arizona,

What are you, stupid? You should've been setting this up years ago. Of course your parents try to make you feel guilty. Guilting hormones, which enable mothers to harangue their children for eternity and beyond, are released in a woman's body during pregnancy. And, of course, men being the Pavlovian creatures they are, learn from their wives after years of training to say, *"It'll kill your mother, but if you don't mind killing your mother, go ahead and do it."*

Here's what you do: Suck it up and go this year. (They already bought the ticket. That's just too much to overcome. They can hold it over your head for the rest of your life.) But next year, stand firm. Say you have to work; you're delivering meals to housebound elderly people; whatever it takes.) This will enable you to start a pattern. You go for two Christmases in a row, then you skip one. Eventually, you taper off to every other Christmas. And that's where you leave it. After all, they did love you and give you money for all those years. It's the least you can do.

P.S. Since you're already obligated this year, try to get with it. Take the Nuisance Lady as an example. She's going to spend the holidays in Miami Beach with Grandma Nuisance, where they'll have a grand old time getting snockered on sloe gin fizzes, rummaging through discount stores, and ripping every other old lady in Grandma Nuisance's retirement community to shreds.

Dead but Not Yet Buried

Dear Nuisance Lady,

Great-Aunt Aggie just died. She never married or had children, so it's up to my brother and me to make all the arrangements. She didn't leave any money to pay for the funeral. She made a killing on the stock market in the early eighties, but it's all gone. God knows what an eighty-four-year-old woman in a one-room apartment was spending her money on, but she was spending it on something.

Anyway, I say there's no point in spending a lot of money on funeral services. She's dead, she didn't have a lot of friends, and I've got kids in college. But my brother says that, out of respect for our late mother (Aunt Aggie was her sister), we've got to do it up right—flowers, a fancy casket, the whole bit. I say she'll never know the difference—have her cremated and sprinkle the ashes in the park (she liked the park). What do you say?

ASHES TO CASH

Dear Ashes,

Oh, she'll know the difference, all right. And so will you. She'll haunt you for the rest of your life. One day you'll be standing in the middle of the A&P and you'll hear a voice: *"So, you can spend $6.49 a pound for chopped sirloin, but you couldn't spend a quarter to give me a decent burial?"* Then you'll hear a second voice: *"How could you embarrass me like that in front of my sister? I'm so ashamed."* Before you know it, you'll be running through the produce section screaming, *"Ma. Ma. I'm sorry, Ma."*

But if the thought of eternal maternal guilt doesn't bother you, go right ahead and have the old broad cremated. Just make sure you go to someone good. One of the Nuisance Lady's cheap cousins got his mother cremated at a discount place. Instead of presenting him with a nice brass urn, they handed him a Hefty bag. I mean, Aunt Essie was a large woman, but come on. The whole family had to go over and help him scatter the "ashes" all over his backyard. It took the whole afternoon.

Has It Been That Long Since *Miami Vice* Went Off the Air?

Dear Nuisance Lady,

My brother's wife is a DEA agent, and every time I see her I want to ram the DEA baseball cap she gave me for Christmas down her throat; then hit her over the head with the DEA coffee mugs she gave me for my birthday. (I won't even tell you what I want to do with the commemorative cuff links.)

She never shuts up about the Dominican drug lords and the Colombian kingpins; not to mention the crackdowns and the big busts. She sounds like Bill Bennett with bad blond highlights.

I happen to believe that drugs should be legalized so that the Colombian kingpins, the Contras, and Good Ole Uncle Sam couldn't continue to get rich off the unfortunate addiction of others.

Every time we're together, we argue about this until she storms off screaming, "I can't sit hear and listen to this Commie crap anymore." Unless I'm at her house; then she shows me the door—the back door (that's the one for Commies). Please tell me how to deal with this fire-breathing, drug-enforcing dragon my brother married.

D(EFINITELY) E(NOUGH) A(LREADY)

◼   ◼   ◼

Dear DEA,

Listen, you little Commie bastard, you're lucky your brother ain't married to Grandpa Nuisance. Then you'd really be in trouble. He sees drug lords and kingpins around every corner—even when he's in temple. He once accused Rabbi Goldfarb of running "cheap rock" out of Chile, whatever that means.

There was a period during the eighties when we thought we were going to have to have him institutionalized. The combination of *Miami Vice* and Nancy Reagan's "Just Say No" campaign was too much for him. He and his friend Sol Weinstein used to dress up like Crockett and Tubbs—an old Crockett and Tubbs—and drive around town in Sol's '74 Lincoln looking for deals going down. (God knows what they were going to do if they actually saw a deal going down.)

He finally calmed down a little in the nineties and the whole family's learned to ignore him whenever he pops out with a "Drugs. They're all dealing drugs."

And you, you little Abbie Hoffman, should do the same. Don't discuss anything that's in any way connected to drug use, abuse, enforcement, etc., with your sister-in-law. Don't even talk about what brand of nasal decongestant works best. And if she brings it up, just ignore, ignore, and ignore some more. Do it for your brother.

P.S. Send the Nuisance Lady all that DEA stuff. Grandpa Nuisance'll love it.

People over Fifty Shouldn't
Play with Dolls

Dear Nuisance Lady,

I own a specialty food store with a partner and friend. We have a good working and personal relationship. There's only one problem: his mother. She's suffering from senility. No, that's not right. She's not suffering from it. She embodies it. Obviously, she can't stay alone, so my partner has started bringing her into the shop every day.

This is having a very bad effect on business because she's scaring the hell out of the customers. She parades around the store in her slip. She insults everyone. The other day she said to a woman buying glazed chestnuts, "They're about the same size as your little titties. Probably as wrinkly too." Then she told our delivery boy, Jesus, that it was "truly amazing" he found his way here from Mexico, since he couldn't find his "way to the top of the Empire State Building on a sunny day."

I don't know what to do. I sympathize with my partner's dilemma. But really, enough is enough. She's going to drive us out of business.

MAD, MAD MOTHER

Dear Mad,

At least she ain't walking around carrying a doll like the Nuisance Lady's aunt Maizy. (In any other family she'd be called Crazy Aunt Maizy, but in the Nuisance Lady's family, insanity is not a distinguishing characteristic.) She and her doll, Daizy, wear matching dresses. An old lady with a doll is freaky enough, but an old lady and her doll wearing the same dress . . . whoa.

Anyway, have a talk with your partner. Be very, very tactful. Say that while you, personally, ADORE his mother and find her offbeat sense of humor absolutely invigorating, Jesus and some of the customers might not share your opinion. Then suggest that perhaps there's no need for both of you to be in the store at the same time. That way he could spend more time at home with Mom. Or you could hire extra help or he could hire a home care professional. There are ways.

P.S. Too bad you didn't say where your store was. The Nuisance Lady would enjoy shopping there, particularly buying cantaloupes.

It's Time to Cut the Cord— the Phone Cord

Dear Nuisance Lady,

I just got off the phone with my sister-in-law. This is the third time today she's called me and it's only 11:30 in the morning. She just had a baby and is a very, very nervous new mother. I already have kids, so she's constantly asking for advice. I don't mind holding her hand a little, but it's getting ridiculous. I have a husband, two kids of my own, and a part-time job. I only have so much time in the day to play Dr. Spock. How can I tell her to lay off a little without hurting her feelings?

NO TIME TODAY

Dear NT,

Please, you think *you* got problems. Grandma and Grandpa Nuisance just got a new dog. The first puppy they've had in twenty years. They're out of their minds. Picture this, a frantic phone call at 2 A.M. *"He looks sick, very sick. He looks green, very green. Come quick."* The Nuisance Lady was halfway uptown in her bathrobe before she realized: (a) She's not a veterinarian, what the hell is she going do? And (b) How could a black Lab look green?

Anyway, some honest, forthright types would tell you, *"Just be open and truthful with her. It's the best way."* Right. You do that and you'll be opening up a big old can of resentment stew. Even if she acts like she understands, she'll secretly be stirring that stew. You weren't there for her in her time of need, blah, blah, smah. The only logical thing to do is to pawn her off on somebody else. Just find one of those women with a baby who loves to talk endlessly, incessantly about their little doopsadoodle. Next time she calls just say, *"You know you should call_____. She's really the expert on burping."*

P.S. The Nuisance Lady was just interrupted by a phone call from Grandma Nuisance, who wanted to know if it would be all right to get undressed in front of the puppy. The burdens some of us must bear.

At Least She's Not Marrying a Geeky White Guy with Big Ears

Dear Nuisance Lady,

I'm a little worried because my daughter has been dating an African American for the last several months. Don't get me wrong, I'm not prejudiced and he's a very nice man. But they're talking marriage, and I'm not sure my daughter knows how difficult a life that would be, particularly for any children they would have. I'm worried my daughter will get angry if I say anything to her about it, but I feel it's my responsibility to speak up. What do you think?

WORRY WART

Dear Worry,

The Nuisance Lady thinks that life is never as easy as we would like it to be. If it were, the Nuisance Lady would be on a beach eating bonbons with a beautiful man beside her, instead of sitting in some crummy studio apartment eating moldy graham crackers answering your letter.

Of course your daughter's life won't be a piece of cake if she marries this man. But whose is? Look at Princess Diana— she married the whitest man in the world. And she's miserable. She makes the Nuisance Lady's aunt Eleanor, with her cataracts and her cross-dressing husband and her daughter in the correctional facility, look like a poster child for Prozac. You should be happy your daughter's getting a nice man. And just remember, easier doesn't always mean better. Or more fun.

P.S. Often when you start a sentence with *"I'm not prejudiced but . . ."* it means that you might be, just a little.

So That's How You Catch Fireflies

Dear Nuisance Lady,

My eighty-five-year-old grandfather is starting to slip a little mentally. Last weekend we had company for lunch. Everything was lovely. I made a delicious salmon with tarragon mustard sauce. After lunch we were sitting by the pool chatting and we look over and there's my grandfather's tushy, bare as on the day he was born. He was changing into a dry bathing suit right in front of everybody. Then the other day he's out in the back-yard with a colander and a peanut butter jar. When I asked him what he was doing, he said he was catching fireflies. In broad daylight. It's two in the afternoon with the sun beating down on his bald head and he's looking for fireflies. I don't know what to do. I don't want to put him in a nursing home, but maybe it's the best thing.

NUTTER BUTTER

Dear Nutter Butter,

All the Nuisance Lady can say is that even though she regu-larly threatens Grandpa Nuisance with a long stay at Sunnydale Rest Home, she would never do it. She's strongly in favor of keeping your old people and your crazy people and your old crazy people at home, where they belong.

So Grandpa's out in the backyard looking for fireflies in his birthday suit! Big deal. Grandpa Nuisance woke the whole house up the other night because he saw SPACE ALIENS in the back-yard. You've never lived until you've chased an old man in polka-dot pj's down a dark country road at three o'clock in the morning.

   P.S. Even though the Nuisance Lady wouldn't send Grandma and Grandpa Nuisance to a nursing home, the Nuisance parents are a different story.

Urban Angst

The Nuisance Lady detests me-ism and victimization, but angst she likes. An angst-ridden hour, even year, here and there can be quite charming. And, let's face it, it's the only shot at profundity most of us have: "The dinginess of these socks reflects the dinginess of my soul."

Okay, so it borders on self-indulgence, but what the hell? Self-indulgence is one of the perks of living in the latter half of the twentieth century. It's just another modern convenience. You get a washer-dryer. You get angst. Besides, it has been very good for the music industry. What is R&B but black angst? Country—white-trash angst. Of course, Latino music's not very "angsty." But that makes sense. You try worrying about the futility of your own existence when you're sitting in the sun, drinking sangría and eating tortillas.

It's Not Just Me and My Shadow Anymore

Dear Nuisance Lady,

I know this may sound crazy, but people are following me. I don't know who these people are, but I know they're there. I can sense them when I'm on the subway or walking down the street. I turn around really quickly to try to catch them, but they're too fast for me. I've tried ducking behind phone booths, hiding behind buses, which, by the way, move too quickly unless you're wearing Rollerblades. Once I even hid in the back of some poor couple from Connecticut's Grand Wagoneer. Boy, were they surprised when they pulled up to their rustic farmhouse and started unloading all the stuff they'd bought at Pottery Barn.

I don't want to tell my parents because they'll just tell me to move back home and live with them for the rest of my life; and my friends will just say I haven't been getting enough sleep lately or something like that. Help, Nuisance Lady, you're the only one I can turn to.

THEY'RE OUT THERE

Dear Out There,

Don't worry, honey, you've come to the right place. First, a few timely questions: Is there any reason for someone to be following you? Are you involved in any mean, mean Russian mob type of activity? Is anyone you're dating involved in any mean, mean Russian mob type of activity? Are there any other signs that someone is stalking you—hang-ups, not-so-funny valentines, etc.? If the answer is yes, then contact the police immediately. But, little tip for you, toots, don't walk into the station house and say, *"Officer, people are following me."*

Now, if you can't think of a reason—even an implausible one—why someone would be following you, this might be a case of *but-people-really-are-following-me* phobia. The Nuisance Lady's dear friend and college roommate Spacy L. A. Lacy suffered from this very same syndrome. She too was diving into bushes and switching cars with people she didn't know. Once she even spent half an hour in a Dimpsy Dumpster (of course, the Nuisance Lady, idiot that she is, was with her at the time).

So you might want to talk to a therapist, perhaps a phone session would be best. (The Nuisance Lady made an in-person appointment for Lacy, but she couldn't go into the building because "they" would've followed her inside.)

P.S. Lacy also believes that absolutely everyone has had a face-lift—even first graders. You should hear her in playgrounds: *"Don't lie to me, kid. I know you've had some work done. You look a lot younger than you did in kindergarten. How do you explain that, huh, huh?"* What are your feelings about plastic surgery? The Nuisance Lady could be onto something here.

If You Have Seven Lives, How Many Deaths Do You Have?

Dear Nuisance Lady,

Lately, I've had several premonitions of my own death. I really, really don't want to die, but I know there's nothing I can do. When your number is up, your number's up, right? I've had a "good run," as they say. I've had thirty fun-filled, adventure-packed years. How can I be more accepting of my fate? Should I tell my friends and family or just let my death come as a surprise?

THE BELL TOLLS FOR ME

Dear Bell,

Listen up, Sarah Bernhardt, you're not dying anytime soon. You people with the death premonitions, it never happens till it happens, usually 100 years and 310 premonitions later. If

Mama Nuisance dropped dead every time she "premoted" it, the Nuisance Lady'd have nothing but a rack of black in her closet, like she does now except there'd be a lot more veils.

Why, just yesterday afternoon Mama Nuisance called to say farewell, again. She had a "feeling" that the plumber—Mr. Manatucci, the nicest man in the world, whom she's known for thirty-five years—was going to hit her over the head with a wrench and spill her brains all over the kitchen floor. Needless to stay, she's still here and the toilet flushes just fine now.

So get out your neon sweat suit and get ready to do fifty or sixty more laps around the track. You've only just finished the warm-up; by the time you're done you'll be sweating like a pig.

And, for your information, thirty years is not a good run; not unless you were a member of a nomadic tribe during the Ice Age. George Bernard Shaw with his ninety-four years of societal acclaim and socialist wit—that was a good run. Picasso with his ninety-two years of Blue periods, and Cubist periods, and painting-all-his-broads-as-giant-genital-chomping-soul-crushing-podheads—that was a good run. Great-Grandma Nuisance with her ninety-seven years of canasta playing, and cheesecake making, and do-you-really-think-she-looks-older-than-me-ing—that was a good run.

Somebody Somewhere Must Have a Really Big Butterfly Collection

Dear Nuisance Lady,

I know this may sound strange, perhaps even trivial, but have you noticed that there are no more butterflies? Maybe I'm imagining this, but it seems there used to be a lot more butterflies around. I never see a butterfly anymore. Where have they all gone?

BUTTERFLY-LESS

Dear Butterfly-less,

Your letter struck a chord with the Nuisance Lady. Visions, visions of summers long past, summers brimming with butterflies skimmed the surface of her consciousness. They led her on one of her rare quests for actual information. (Ordinarily, calling professionals, any type of professional, is something the Nuisance Lady despises and seeks to avoid at all costs.) She called observatories, conservancies, laboratories, and spoke with numerous observers, conservers, preservers, etc. And she came to one conclusion: People who devote their lives to flora, fauna, and bugs are nice, very nice. Everyone the Nuisance Lady spoke with was just lovely.

Anyway, it seems that the butterfly population has in fact been declining in recent years. This is due to a variety of factors, including drought, development, and disease. Butterflies need water and wildlife, wild shrubbery anyway, in order to thrive and lay their chrysalises down. They also need fields. Green, open fields. (Go find a field these days, one that hasn't been multiplexed.)

P.S. Here's the difference between a writer and a conserva-
tionist, a person who cares about butterflies. Upon reading this
column a colleague of the Nuisance Lady's said, *"That butterfly
thing is good. You could start a national friggin' save-the-butterfly
campaign.*

BUTTERFLIES AREN'T FREE. *Somethin' like that. Great
symbolism. Make great T-shirts. Then you could embezzle all the
money. Funnel it through a Swiss bank account. Move to South America.
They gotta have some real friggin' butterflies left down there."*

Stay out of Museums, If You Know What's Good for You

Dear Nuisance Lady,

Yesterday I went to a museum and it depressed the hell out
of me; staring at all those Renoirs, Rossettis, and Matisses made
me want to weep. You see, I'm a beer salesman, and while I'm
handsomely compensated for my labors and get all kinds of free
perks like going to the MTV Music Awards party, I can't help
feeling that my life is less than what it should be. I mean I don't
create anything great, anything that grabs humanity by the
throat and lifts its spirits. When I die, I will not be able to say
that mankind was enriched one iota by my presence here. Can
you think of anything to cheer me up, Nuisance Lady? I'm really
feeling horrible about this.

CERTAINLY NOT MATISSE

Dear Matisse,

The Nuisance Lady is only on her first cup of coffee, so it's a little early for grabbing anyone by the throat. But a little tip for you, sweets: We can't all be Matisse. In fact, practically none of us can. There are, what, four or five Matisses running around in the world at any given time? What are the chances you would have been born one of them? Think about it. Besides, you do enrich people's lives. You make them a little drunker on Friday night. Personally, the Nuisance Lady often finds a nice cold one incredibly enriching. Try to remember what the Nuisance Lady's great-uncle Abe from the old country would've said in a situation like this: *"To hell with Matisse, thank God my house hasn't burned down today, and I still have some goats standing in the field."*

There's Nothing to Fear but Fear Itself; Isn't That Enough?

Dear Nuisance Lady,

I have fears. Lots of them. Every time I eat something, I'm scared it's been poisoned by some maniac with a grudge against cookies. Every time I watch TV I'm afraid that I won't be able to stop and my life'll pass by in a blur of sit-coms. When I walk down the street, I'm scared that an out-of-control air conditioner will fall from a window and hit me on the head. I'm scared that I'll become a suburban man with a minivan, mowing the lawn, barbecuing with the neighbors, and lusting after the teenage cheerleader next door. Or that I'll die a lonely, old, urban man with lots of cats, drinking wine from a jug, and eating soup from a can. I know this may sound silly, but these fears are literally keeping me awake at night.

FRAIDY CAT

Dear Fraidy,

It could be worse, you could die alone—without cats. Dying with cats is one thing, but dying without cats . . .

Let's try a little role playing. (The Nuisance Lady loves role playing.) Tonight you'll go to bed as a little fraidy cat, but you'll wake up as UNFLAPPABLE MAN. (Or you could be Unflappable Mouse, Ant, Dog, whatever you prefer.) Anyway, UNFLAPPABLE MAN can bite into an oatmeal cookie without fear. He can walk down the street with his head held high, not scanning the sky. He can stare a Sony Trinitron right in the remote—and not turn it on. He can leap into a second date without being bound. He can even go to the pound and adopt a stray. He simply cannot be flapped. And that's that.

If that doesn't work, you can always move to a rural area with no TVs, cheerleaders, or minivans for miles around, grow all your own food, get a dog, and buy lots of wineglasses. But that would take an awfully long time—and life's much shorter than that.

There Is No Hidden Meaning

Dear Nuisance Lady,

What am I doing with my life? I can't tell you how much I would appreciate an answer to that question. I have a so-so job with not much room for advancement. I have a guy that I "see" but don't really love. I go to the gym and futilely climb a StairMaster day in and day out. I do lots and lots of crunches too. But the sought-after "six-pack" continues to elude me. And I'm no spring chicken anymore. Is there anything I can do to make my life more meaningful?

GETTING WEARY WEARING THAT SAME OLD DRESS

Dear Weary,

You know what the difference is between you and everyone else? NOTHING. Wise up, sweets. You are suffering from nothing more than postmodern, end-of-the-century, urban angst. This, as a very wise poli-sci professor once explained to the Nuisance Lady, comes from too much leisure time combined with inflated expectations fueled by the mass media. Back in the days of wine and roses, whenever those were, people didn't expect to be happy or have "meaningful" lives because they were too busy scavenging for turnips in the dirt or working twenty hours a day in a cotton mill. It wasn't until the twenties with the advent of the motorcar, that people began to feel a vague gnawing emptiness.

Stop expecting life to be so damned meaningful, toots, and you'll be much better off. Also, the Nuisance's Lady's gym-boy friend, Frederico, says it's almost impossible for women to get "six-packs" because they have a built-in layer of "insulation" (fat) around the middle to protect potential babies. In other words, in order to get one, you'd have to eat nothing, quit your job, stop socializing, and "crunch" all day long. Forget about it.

Instant Anything

Dear Nuisance Lady,

You know what occurred to me the other day as I was walking past a Pottery Barn? We have become an artificial "insta-society" in which countless façades can be effortlessly erected, disassembled, and new ones put in their place for only a few hundred dollars. You want that light, airy "country French" look, just go to a Crate & Barrel. You want that East Village "urban angst" look, there's an Urban Outfitters around the corner. You want a kitchen with that "warm cozy" feel to it, there's a Williams-Sonoma waiting for you. Nothing has to be cultivated anymore. Nothing has to be nurtured anymore. (You don't even have to spend a lot of money to get it anymore.) What's going to become of this society, in which everything is instantly available at a low cost with little or no effort? How long before it is strangled by its own torpidness, before its inert corps starts rotting from the inside?

INSTA-THOUGHT

Dear Insta,

It could go on for a long time. Look at those big fat guys who eat fried mozzarella sticks and smoke cigars all day. A lot of them live forever. You can't kill em with a stick. Your observations about our postmodern culture are quite correct—not that original, but quite correct. You know who's responsible for it, don't you? Ralph Lauren. The former Mr. Lifshitz or whatever his name was. He started it all with his polo shirts and his look-like-a-Connecticut-WASP-even-if-you've-never-played-field-hockey-or-been-near-Nantucket-in-your-life marketing campaign. His name is definitely at the top of the "Responsible for the Decline of Western Civilization" list.

Nothing Doing

Dear Nuisance Lady,

I don't do anything and I don't want to. Do you find that strange? You see, I *used* to do a zillion things a day. I was running from morning till night. I had two jobs. I took classes. I went to the gym. I was buff. I had a boyfriend. But for some reason I stopped doing things, one by one. I asked myself if I really needed to do this or that and the answer was always "No, not really." So now I have no jobs, take no classes. Lost the boyfriend and am back to my bony, decidedly "unbuff" self.

Here's the strange part: I've never been happier. I wake up when I want to. I eat a breakfast burrito at any time of the day. I spend hours looking out the window watching my street. I've read all of *Sexus, Plexus,* and *Nexus,* as well as *The Brothers K* and significant portions of *Finnegans Wake.* Time has, to use an ubiquitous cliché, lost all meaning. (My watch is somewhere under the bed, I think. And I haven't bought batteries for my clock in months.)

The only dark clouds on my ever-expanding horizon are friends and family who constantly harass me with their well-intentioned entreaties to "resume" my life or their not-so-well-intentioned threats to have me institutionalized. I love them all dearly, but they just don't understand how happy and serene my life has become. Please give me some meaningful advice.

THE DO-NOTHING GIRL

Dear Do-Nothing,

Hey, honey, you left a few details out of your letter, like how the hell you're paying for all this doing-nothing. If you're being supported by anyone, such as Mommy and Daddy, they have every right to ask you to get off your unbuffed butt and get a job. But if by some weird contortion of fate, you have an independent income from, say, a long-dead aunt who bought lots of Coca-Cola stock, that's a different story entirely.

Even if the Nuisance Lady can kind of understand how someone could be happy reading the classics and eating burritos all day, she also knows that society—a few Generation X movies notwithstanding—does not really tolerate people of leisure. So, you might want to consider getting at least a part-time job. That will still leave you plenty of time for other stuff. And let's face it—staring out the window of your apartment is a lot better than staring out the window of some sanitarium.

I'll Cut Off More Than Those Shorts, Honey

Dear Nuisance Lady,

My husband and I recently moved from the city to the suburbs. We did this so we could afford to have kids, and so these kids could have a lawn. Well, now we have them: one kid and a lawn. The problem is that I'm bored, bored, bored out of my bean. There's nothing here but an Ace Hardware, and a Dunkin' Donuts. I'm used to a bustling metropolis full of bistros, boutiques, and ballets. What can I do to make this banishment to the 'burbs more bearable?

GOING CRAZY ON A CUL-DE-SAC

P.S. I tried hiring a baby-sitter (a local college girl) so I could get into the city a couple of times a week, but she's unreliable and my newborn doesn't travel well.

Dear Cul-de-Sac,

Have you lost your mind? You don't hire some little hotpants college girl to take care of your kid. She'll parade around in front of your husband in cutoffs and crop tops, and before you know it, you'll be back in the city all right—at the office of a good divorce lawyer. Hire some big fat Romanian woman with hairs growing out of her moles.

Furthermore, as Mama Nuisance used to say on many a rainy day, *"Bored Shmored, we'll put a Brillo pad in your hand, little Missy, and see how fast you get unbored."* Just because you're in suburbia with a baby doesn't mean you have to sit around watching trash TV and eating French bread pizzas. Find something fun to do in the house. Origami, papier-mâché, tiramisù. Take pictures of the tile in your bathroom. (Actually, the Nuisance Lady's friend Rosalee did that and the pictures ended up in some gallery in Soho as part of a "Salute to the Household Object" exhibit.) Don't forget, if you get really desperate there's always catalog shopping.

I May Be Rhoda Morgenstern, but the Chick Next Door Definitely Ain't Mary Richards

Dear Nuisance Lady,

I think the woman next door is a hooker. Okay, I live in a very nice building, so maybe she's an "escort." But something funny's going on over there. Men are coming, and I mean that literally—the walls are very thin—and going all the time, at all hours of the day and night. (And not handsome young men either—graying, balding business types.) When I asked her what she did for a living, she said she was a consultant. Yeah, I know what she consults all right. What can I do about this? I've made lots of complaints, but I think she's bribing the landlord or something.

APARTMENT OF ILL REPUTE

Dear A.I.R.,

Look at it this way, it could be worse. You could live in between a gay serial killer and a very, very bad sax player like the Nuisance Lady does. The gay serial killer, she's not 100 percent sure about, but he's got a lot of guys going in and none coming out, so you've got to wonder.

Anyway, back to your Rear Window. Of course she's a hooker. Believe me, honey, nobody enjoys having sex with middle-aged bald guys that much. Unfortunately, if she's bribing people there's not much you can do about it. There's an old Chinese proverb: *Money talks and lets hookers walk.* Actually, you could try calling up the vice squad and telling them that you've seen celebrities going in and out. Seems like everybody loves a high-profile bust these days.

Pick Me Up, Please

Dear Nuisance Lady,

Because I walk with a cane, it's almost impossible for me to get a cab. I stand on the corner and watch the taxis whiz on by. I can actually get around quite well and wouldn't be any more trouble than someone without a cane. My sister says the cabbies are probably worried about lawsuits. Perhaps you could ask some cab driver of your acquaintance what the problem is.

CANE THOSE CABBIES

P.S. Little do they know I'm a good tipper.

Dear Cane,

You're lucky you're not a young black man with a baby, a bag of groceries, a cat carrier, and a cane. You'd be there until the groceries spoiled, the cat died, and the kid graduated from college.

The Nuisance Lady was, in fact, able to track down two cab drivers of her acquaintance: Hammar the Good and his brother Bammar the Bad. Hammar says, and the Nuisance Lady quotes, *"I always stop to pick up everybody. Everybody. They got no money. They got no clothes. They got skin disease. It no matter. I take them where they want to go."*

But his brother Bammar says, and the Nuisance Lady quotes again, *"I don't have time for no stinking canes. I be there for three stinking hours with stinking canes. Stinking crutches. Stinking pregnant woman. No stinking time. Time is money. Money no stinking."* Unfortunately, there are a lot more Bammars out there than Hammars.

So the Nuisance Lady can only suggest that you move to

London. Now that's a city for cab connoisseurs. What we call cab drivers and what they call cab drivers shouldn't even be called the same thing. The Nuisance Lady has fond memories of a cabbie named Colin who took her and Nana Nuisance all over that town. They started at the Tower of London. (For some reason Nana had a strong desire to see the place where they cut off people's heads.) Colin knew more history than most Ph.D.s and was also a good little shopper. He helped Nana pick out souvenirs for her friends Fritzi, Mitzi, and Mrs. Di Angelo. He even fried us up some fish 'n' chips in the glove compartment.

P.S. The only other thing the Nuisance Lady can say is—car service.

Help, I've Fallen into the Abyss of Time and I Can't Get Up

Dear Nuisance Lady,

I'm obsessed with the passage of time. It started when I read some stupid article that calculated how many minutes the average person will spend doing certain things in his lifetime, like brushing his teeth (44,750), or dancing around the house naked (18,201), or looking for a parking space (71,393). Ever since then I've been hypersensitive to all things temporal. I'll be standing on line for the movies and I'll start thinking, "Eight and a half minutes, man. That's almost nine minutes of my life gone just like that. I could've been doing something else with that nine minutes." Or else I'll be at the movies thinking, "171 minutes. I can't believe I'm wasting 171 minutes on this lousy movie." Asking for my money back just doesn't seem to cut it. I mean, what's a few bucks compared to the big hourglass of life trickling away?

How do I get this obsession under control? It's really starting to affect my life. The other day in a meeting my boss yelled at me for constantly looking at my watch, and I won't even tell you what my girlfriend said when she caught me checking the clock in the middle of sex.

BIG BEN

Dear Ben,

Interesting. It seems like people should be spending a lot more time brushing their teeth and dancing around the house naked and a lot less time looking for a parking space.

You say you're obsessed with time—hours, minutes, seconds. Wait till you start sitting on the sofa with a stopwatch trying to split those seconds into milliseconds. The Nuisance Lady once spent an entire weekend suspended in time trying to do just that.

It started on a Paris street corner when the innocent Nuisance Lady stopped to ask a stranger the time. The stranger, being always-and-ever-so-obligingly French, replied: *"Est-ce que j'ai l'air d'un Rolex?"* Which, roughly translated, means he pointed to his forehead and said, "Do you see Rolex written here, honey?"

Suddenly, Orson Wellesian visions of official time tellers

danced in the Nuisance Lady's head—on every street corner of every city, town, and village—austere, nimble creatures in gray leotards, kind of like mice in a Martha Graham production.

As you strolled along on a Saturday afternoon, stopping to look at a pair of khaki shorts in a Banana Republic window, there they'd be—dangling imaginary pocket watches on the end of imaginary chains, chanting: "Tick tock, tick tock . . ." You could destroy an entire civilization like that. Much cheaper than nuclear arms. (Blofeld's got nothing on the Nuisance Lady.)

Just remember, Big Sweet Ben, time marches on, until you run out; then it stops. It's inevitable. And never ask Pierre for the time of day.

30 Is the Yuckiest Number

Dear Nuisance Lady,

I do not believe this is happening to me. In less than seventy-two hours I'm going to be thirty. I can't eat. I can't sleep. I can't function at work. It's the only thing I can think about. It's just there like this enormous, unyielding, Mount Rushmore type of thing. I feel like my life has just become one giant "Schoolhouse Rock" song: *What's 3 times 10? What's 5 times 6? What's someone who's 30 with a so-so job and no marriage prospects? LOSER.*

Help! I'm so desperate I'm ready to enroll in Devry or Apex or one of those technical schools you see on TV and become an air conditioner–repair person. Then I'm going to move to

Alaska, where the ratio of men to women is 100,000 to 1 or something like that.

ALMOST THERE

Dear Almost,

Ahh, the Nuisance Lady remembers it well—the big 3-O panic. (Don't you hate the way people say that, the big 3-O, with such emphasis on the O?)

Okay, this is what it's like turning thirty. You wake up, you make coffee, you go to work. You endure some juvenile ribbing from friends and colleagues, a little "if only" sighing from your mother, and then it's over. If you want to make the best of it, try something new and fun—something that you've always wanted to do. (The Nuisance Lady tried fencing on her thirtieth birthday, something she'd always wanted to do. Although it's not as much fun as you might think—they don't wear those cool all-white outfits anymore, just regular workout clothes. And you don't get to draw first blood—there's a little electronic beep that goes off when you "touch" someone.)

Anyway, as far as your life goes, don't let yourself become one of those panicky, whining, Oh-my-God-I'm-not-married-yet type of broads. (A blight on the semiflawless surface of the female sex if ever there was one.) Look at it this way: The later you get married, the less chance you'll get sick of him before death or senility sets in. As far as your career goes, if you're not happy with your job, look for a new one. *Hello.*

P.S. Maybe it's because you're worried about turning thirty or maybe you're just not the sharpest tool in the shed, but there's probably not a big demand for air conditioner–repair people in Alaska.

Kids
(God's Little Gumdrops)

The Nuisance Lady likes kids in their raw form before the parents get hold of them. And today's parents, the yuppie parents in all their equally appalling variations, are the worst. Deafened by a pair of Dr. Spock ears, they aren't the least bit distressed by their children's constant consumer ranting, "Buy me, Buy me, Buy me." Does any kid even need one Death Ray of Mass Destruction, let alone ten? We ought to take a cue from the French. They take their kids out, plunk them down in cafés, and expect them to act like normal people. No ordering off the kiddie menu for little Pierre and Marie. If you ask the Nuisance Lady, there ought to be a lot less *Sesame Street* watching and a lot more café sitting going on. And Christmas should come only once every four years—like the Olympics. And no kid should get a present that costs more than a seven-course meal at McDonald's.

Can You Say Penis and Vagina? You're Going to Have To

Dear Nuisance Lady,

I think it's time to tell my son the facts of life. He's five and he's already starting to ask questions like, "If I rub my willy woo real hard, will I get a baby?" My mother, however, says that he's still way too young to be told about sex. What do you think?

IS IT TIME

Dear Time,

What are you, crazy? You're going to take advice about sex education from your mother? Were you so enlightened and edified growing up?

Of course you should tell your son about sex, if you think he's ready. It'll be fun. You'll make little drawings. (You could even buy that cool book with the big black letters and the little naked people.) You'll get to say the words *penis* and *vagina* more times than a gynecologist and a proctologist do in a week. It'll be great.

Your letter is bringing back fond memories of first grade: all the little girls standing by the water fountain and Cassie Krakowski explaining how our daddies had stuck their penises in our mommies' vaginas. All the other little chickadees squealing, *"Oooh, gross, my mommy and daddy would never do that."* The little Nuisance Lady thinking, *"Sounds like fun. Can't wait to grow up and try it."*

P.S. Willy woo, huh? Love the names that families come up with for genitalia? The Nuisance Lady's friend Patsy still refers to her pookalakie. Ridiculous. Everyone knows it's a chi-chi. Even worse, the Nuisance Lady once dated a guy who had a King Do Do.

Cinderella as a Second Wife

Dear Nuisance Lady,

I detest my stepchildren. The loathsome little creatures sit around the house all day doing nothing. My stepson, who is twenty-seven, is supposedly working on his "screenplay," but I've never ever seen him actually write anything. He just sits at his computer all day long playing video games and talking to other idiots on the Net. My stepdaughter, twenty-three, can't work because she has an eating disorder of some sort and work would be too physically taxing. All she does is sleep all day and drop pumpkin seeds all over the house.

My husband says he doesn't want to pressure his children and wants them to have all the advantages he never did. I've tried to say something to them, but they think of me as "that gold-digging little bitch Dad dug out of the sandbox." I love my husband and our lifestyle, but I don't know how much more of this I can take.

No Cinderella Story

Dear Cinderella,

You young broads marry these old guys in the middle of their midlife crises and you expect it to be all Beluga and bikini waxes at Bergdorf's. Wake up and smell wife number one's perfume. What do you think you're getting, nine times out of ten, when you marry a man who dumps his wife of twenty-odd years for a broad who was in kindergarten the year he graduated law school? How many times does the Nuisance Lady have to say it? All you young broads, listen up: Buy a pack of Bic disposable razors for $1.39 and stick with a guy your own age. In the long run you'll be much better off.

Now, toots, since you've already gotten yourself into this situation . . . tell your husband that, divorce guilt or no divorce guilt, the little layabouts have got to get jobs. (Hopefully, you have one yourself.) Then, once they get these jobs they've got to move out of the house. Children past a certain age are just not meant to live in the same house with their parents.

Finally, even if your stepchildren are the devil's own, always, always treat them kindly and never try to stop your husband from spending time or money on them. Kids are not as easy to get rid of as first wives. Should've thought of that before you married him, sweets.

If This Is High School, How Come It Has So Many Lows?

Dear Nuisance Lady,

You have no idea how ugly my nose is. It's so horrible. It's huge and it curves to the right. I think it's the only reason I didn't get the lead in the school play. We're doing *West Side Story* except with cool music, you know, like Bush and Fiona Apple. That bitch Zoe Kadan with the perfect nose got it instead. I keep telling my mother that there's no way I can be an actress with this nose, but she says there's nothing wrong with my nose and that when I'm older I'll appreciate it. Help me,

Nuisance Lady. How can I convince her that if she doesn't let me have a nose job, my life'll be ruined?

NOBODY NOSE

Dear Nose,

Your charming letter reminds the Nuisance Lady of her high school days, when that bitch Samantha Chapell got to play the shrew in the senior class production of *The Taming of the Shrew*. Can you believe that? Who would've made a better shrew than the Nuisance Lady? Samantha only got it because of her shameless and relentless sucking-up to Ms. Rappaport, the drama teacher: *I'll carry that to your car for you, Ms. Rappaport. I'll get you another diet Sprite, Ms. Rappaport.* (Don't you worry though; the sight of the Nuisance Lady and Samantha's so-called boyfriend, Chris Goodson, at Billy Falardi's Halloween party wiped that saccharine smile right off her face.)

Oops, the Nuisance Lady just had a little attack of high school. Back to you and your no-doubt-perfectly-lovely nose. Your mother, who by the way is probably supposed to pay for this nose job, has a very good point—our tastes change dramatically after high school. So while the thought of some hideous, overly pinched, Jersey girl nose might be appealing to you now, it will most certainly lose its attractions as you ripen into the full flower of womanhood. (The Nuisance Lady's had way, way too much coffee.)

Forget about the nose job for now. If you still want it when you can pay for it, go right ahead. And don't worry about not getting the part of Maria in *West Side Story*. It's stupid. How Natalie Wood could have sung that "I Feel Pretty" song and kept a straight face, you gotta wonder.

Stay Away from the Fake Mutton Chops

Dear Nuisance Lady,

A few months ago my wife and I took our kids to one of those medieval fairs in Jersey. You know, the kind with the fake jousting and the fake maidens serving fake mutton chops and everybody's throwing fake flowers in the air.

Anyway, everybody had a good time dancing, eating the fake mutton, and throwing the fake flowers up in the air. It's all hunky-dory except since we got back my eight-year-old's decided he's a knight of the friggin Round Table. He makes us call him Sir Frankie Jr. and he wears some tinfoil getup around the house all the time. The kids at school are starting to make fun of him because he's saying things like "Give me not that green marker. It's the red one I seek."

At first it was kind of funny, but now it's starting to get on my nerves. I want to bust up the Round Table with a good spanking but my wife says we've got to let him express himself. What do you think?

KOOKY KID THINKS HE'S IN CAMELOT

Dear Kooky Kid,

Somehow, Sir, one can well imagine that your home is no Camelot. However, the fact that your extraordinarily imaginative and intelligent son chooses to perceive it as such is cause for celebration, not spankings. In this age of Sega-addicted little automatons, you should get down on your hands and knees and thank the gods for a child with such a keen sense of the chimerical. Why, the Nuisance Lady herself spent much of her fifth and sixth years as Princess Ashanti of All the Egypts, both Upper and Lower. She can well remember saying things like *"Corn-flakes, cornflakes. Princess Ashanti does not eat cornflakes for break-fast."* And, of course, who could forget Mama Nuisance's raspy Maxwell Housed and Marlboroed response. *"Sorry, toots, we're all out of nectar and manna this morning."*

Can Fish Be Drowned?

Dear Nuisance Lady,

Maybe you can help settle a family dispute. My husband and I have decided to get our son a pet because it will teach him about responsibility and caring, blah, blah, blah. The problem is that we can't agree on what type of pet. My husband wants to get him an ordinary, everybody-has-one dog, and I want to get him a splendid aquarium filled with a breathtaking array of brightly colored tropical fish. Who's right? Don't forget you don't have to walk an aquarium and it doesn't make a mess on the Persian rug.

PETS ON PARK AVENUE

Dear Pets,

Fish. The Nuisance Lady hates fish. Forget the fish. Yeah, yeah, everybody says they have a soothing effect. So what? If the Nuisance Lady wants to be soothed, she'll buy a bottle of Southern Comfort, not a slimy little goldfish. Can your kid hug an aquarium, the cold glass and steel edges pressing up against his little cheek? Can he take it to the park to play with the other aquariums? Toss it a Frisbee? Get the kid a retriever, for God's sake.

At-Home Religious Wars

Dear Nuisance Lady,

I'm a Jewish girl from Kew Gardens and my husband is a WASP from deep Connecticut. Before our son, Alex, was born we agreed to "expose" him to both faiths and then allow him to make his own decision when he felt ready. Well, that is what we said, but since Alex has reached the "age of reason," both my husband and I seem to have lost our minds. Between Sunday school and Hebrew school, he doesn't have any free time. The other day, Rosh Hashanah, the poor kid was like a relay baton, with my husband and I passing him off from temple to church, rabbi to reverend. I know this isn't fair to my little *bubbeleh*, but neither my husband nor I want to give in. Please help, Nuisance Lady; we both agreed that we'd abide by whatever you decided. (We figured it was better than flipping a coin.)

WIFE OF A WONDER BREAD WASP

Dear Wife,

Does the word SELFISH mean anything to you? (And the Nuisance Lady doesn't mean the thing you're not allowed to eat, little rugelach.) Obviously, the "agreement" you and your husband reached needs to be revised. First, you should curtail little Alex's "exposure" to both religions. Hey, the kid needs a life. This means he goes to temple one Saturday a month and church one Sunday a month or something like that.

Second, you should alternate holidays: Celebrate Christmas, not Hanukkah; then Passover, not Easter. If you give the kid a choice between Christmas and Hanukkah, he'll make a beeline for the Christmas tree, knocking over the menorah on the way. (Christmas is more "fun" and involves more presents in a shorter period of time.) Last, and most important, neither one of you should ever, ever denigrate the faith of the other in front of the little lamb.

Skating in Very Thin Sequined Tights

Dear Nuisance Lady,

My sister took my seven-year-old son ice skating a couple of times this year and he really loved it. So now she wants to give him ice skating lessons as a birthday present. My husband, however, says "no way." He says ice skating is for girls, and he doesn't want his son doing anything so sissylike. I think he's being ridiculous and Archie Bunker–like. Who's right?

PROUD TO HAVE A SON IN SKATES

Dear Proud,

This is a tough one. If it was ballet, the Nuisance Lady would be with you 100 percent. Have you seen those guys in tights? (Although the Nuisance Lady must admit she was very disappointed when she recently learned that male dancers wear protective clothing, which makes objects appear deceptively larger.)

Anyway, skating is a different story. While the Nuisance Lady deplores your husband's homophobic, sexist attitude, she has an equal if not greater disdain for the costumes worn by male ice skaters. Can you honestly say that you would want your son parading around in a skintight, purple-sequined, pirate costume? If he's performing at the Purple Banana, okay. But on *CBS Sports*? Eh, let the kid take some lessons, but if he starts talking about his salchows, put a stop to it.

Stupid As They Wanna Be

Dear Nuisance Lady,

My young nieces and nephews paid me a visit recently. I haven't seen them in quite some time, but I have to say that I was shocked to discover what ignoramuses they had become. They know absolutely nothing about any given subject. I doubt if they could even tell you what state they are living in, let alone its capital. They do nothing but sit around and play video games, eat strange foods, and stare into space; that is, of course, when they're not watching TV. I think it's rather lax of my brother to permit this sort of sloth. However, when I mentioned this to him, he simply shrugged his shoulders and said, "Kids today. That's just the way they are." Is this true or is my brother just lazy?

UNCLE OF THE UNEDUCATED MASSES

■　　　■　　　■

Dear Uncle,

The Nuisance Lady is of the firm belief that ignorance and indolence should be beaten and starved out of children if necessary. More parents should follow the example set by a very wise professor the Nuisance Lady once knew. Every night when the professor and all of his nine children, legitimate and otherwise, sat down to dinner, he would ask them each a question. The subjects varied, anything from mathematics to modern art. After a second wrong answer, the child was forced to leave the table without supper. Once, some smart aleck remarked that the stupid ones must be really skinny. *"There are no stupid ones,"* the wise professor replied.

Help, My Washer's Stuck on the God Cycle

Dear Nuisance Lady,

Recently my six-year-old son asked me what God was. Being a secular yet spiritual soul, I told him that God was an essence that was all around us, in everything. His imaginative yet impetuous young mind decided to take this definition literally, and he now really believes that God is "everywhere." As a result I can't use any of my household appliances. Every time I try to turn on the washing machine or garbage disposal, he starts crying and screaming, "Stop it, Mommy. You're hurting God." I've tried explaining to him that God is not corporeal and cannot be "hurt" like people can, but he doesn't believe me. What can I do? If I have to do one more load of laundry by hand I'm going to scream.

No Deity in the Dishwasher

Dear Dishwasher,

You seem like an eloquent, erudite woman, and this, toots, is the *essence* of your problem. In other words, can the cerebral conversations with your kid. Explain this God-thing to him in terms he can understand. Tell him that God is like a superhero or a Mighty Morphin Power Ranger—nothing, not even a May-tag, can harm him. Next time you do a load of laundry, stop it in midcycle, and show him that there are no God-guts splattered inside.

P.S. Look on the sunny side: In a week he'll be on to something else, and you'll have a cute-kid story for life. When the Nuisance Lady was little, she thought God was Richard Nixon in a pink chiffon evening gown. (Hey, it was the combination of Watergate and the Miss America pageant.)

Bold, Bold Boys

Dear Nuisance Lady,

I'm appalled by my kids' behavior whenever we go shopping. They never stop with the "I-want-this" and "I-want-that." I certainly didn't teach them to act like that. What can I do so I don't wind up with spoiled, materialistic little brats?

Brat Packed

■　　■　　■

Dear Packed,

You can do what the Nuisance Lady's friend Flanagan's father used to do. But you have to do it with a brogue, or else it won't work. Pick up the phone and say, *"Oh, yes, Mr. Collins, from the Special School for Bold Boys, you've got a van in the neighborhood. You'll be here in five minutes."* Then, after much twinging and tweaking and I'll-be-good, you say, *"Well, Mr. Collins, I think we'll hold off for a while, but don't go very far."* The trick is to make them think that that van is just circling the neighborhood waiting, at any given moment, to take them to the Special School for Bold Boys (or Girls). If only Mama Nuisance had known about that school. (For the Nuisance Lady's horrible sisters, of course.)

The Prettiest Girl in the Class Never Lasts

Dear Nuisance Lady,

My problem is that I'm really, really ugly. I'm so ugly that no guy would even look at me or think about asking me out. My mother says I'm just going through my awkward stage and I'll grow out of it soon. But I don't believe her. I know I'll be ugly forever. Why can't I be like Amanda Adams? She's the prettiest girl in my class. Everything about her is perfect: Her hair, her body, even her feet are perfect. Even ninth and tenth grade guys want to go out with her. I'm so miserable. If I don't grow up to look like a supermodel, I'll die.

GRUESOME

Dear Gruesome,

If you don't grow up to look like a supermodel, the only thing that'll happen to you is that you'll go to college. And you won't marry a rock star. These are good things. A college degree you'll have for life, a rock-star husband you'd have for two months.

Listen up, the Nuisance Lady's going to tell you a story of two girls. One, Holly Hardaway, was just like Amanda Adams. The prettiest girl in the eighth grade. (Who, of course, had an alliterative name, because the prettiest girl in junior high always has an alliterative name.) Anyway, this Holly Hardaway was hot stuff; even eleventh graders were knocking at her locker.

But, unfortunately—as with all fruits, flowers, and girls that bloom too early—time was not kind to her. Talk about hard-looking; even Mama Nuisance's new industrial-strength, drop-dead-red acrylic nails don't look like that.

The second girl was, in fact, the Nuisance Lady's not-so-much-younger sister Mo. You should've seen that girl when she was twelve: fat little face, hair like Richard Simmons's, more pimples than a goose flying over the Arctic Circle. Today, only a few short years later, she is a flawless-skinned, long-auburn-haired, little-black-dress-wearing knockout. And the same thing will happen to you, toots. Just remember, better later than in the seventh grade.

P.S. When you get older, you'll realize that there's a big beauty line. Cindy Crawford's in front of you and Roseanne's in back of you. And that ain't such a bad thing.

Put Your Kid on a Leash, He'll Come Back and Kill You in Your Sleep

Dear Nuisance Lady,

My husband and I bought our fifteen-year-old son a beeper. We thought it would make it easier to keep tabs on him. However, he got very upset when we gave it to him and absolutely refuses to carry it. He says it's like we want to spy on him all the time. What do you think?

BEEP HOME

Dear Beep,

Uhh, of all the twisted things the Nuisance Lady's heard—and she's heard plenty—that is the most twisted. The poor kid, you're making him star in "Beavis and Butthead Do *1984*." What's next, you send him off to the glue factory like the poor horses in *Animal Farm*? Do you expect to be able to beep him for the rest of his life? *"Suzy, will you marry . . . ?"* Beep. *"So, Mr. ———, what makes you qualified for this job?"* Beep. Beep.

Kids are not cattle. They should not be forced to wear leashes when they're little. Or carry beepers when they're big. Hell, cattle shouldn't even be forced to carry beepers: *"Hey, Fred up at the slaughterhouse has been beeping you all morning."*

Give the beeper to your husband instead. Kids and cattle shouldn't be forced to carry beepers, but husbands . . .

For God's Sake, Even Mickey Mouse Is Married

Dear Nuisance Lady,

My family's going to Disney World for vacation and I don't want to go. I'm sixteen and I think that's old enough to stay home by myself, but my parents say I can't stay alone until next year. Don't you think they're being mean and hateful? I'll have a horrible time without any of my friends, just following my parents around EPCOT, and taking my stupid little brothers on Space Mountain. Tell them, Nuisance Lady. Maybe they'll listen to you.

NO MORE MICKEY

Dear Mickey,

Honey, honey, honey. You think you got it tough, try going to Disney World with your family when you're over thirty—and not married. *"Look over there, it's Daisy."* Isn't she *married to Donald? "And Mickey."* He's married too. *"Isn't that a beautiful orange tree?"* Yeah, it's married to the lemon tree *across the way. "If it's such a Small World, you'd think you wouldn't have any trouble finding a husband. Even in 20,000* Leagues Under *the Sea that girl found a husband. Better the pirate should kill me with his sword than I should live another day without you being married. Never-never land—maybe we'll hold your reception there. Excuse me, Mr. Keystone Cop, have you met my granddaughter?"*

Go, go now, when you're young and the worst they can do is bust you for smoking a joint on Space Mountain. Tomorrow Land ain't no Mr. Toad's Wild Ride. Trust the Nuisance Lady.

P.S. The keystone cops actually have the power to arrest you and take you to the keystone jail. Spitting, they give you a warning. But strangling, they throw the book at you.

Intoxicated, Liberated, Dissipated—
The Fine Line

BEWARE THE VICELESS. Not having any vices, not wanting to smoke or drink—or even eat—anything. Or worse, being tempted to smoke, drink, or eat something and having the self-discipline to refrain—all the time—it just ain't normal. Sober people are scary. You never know what they'll do. Or rather, they always know what they did; and even worse, they always remember what you've done.

Don't believe them when they tell you that having that extra glass of carrot juice or taking that last run down the mountain is a vice. Skiing is not a vice. Vegetables are not vices. There are only three legitimate vices: Drinking, Smoking, and Some Kinds of Sex. Well, maybe four, if you count Gambling—but, as anyone who's ever been to Vegas can tell you, that's not exactly a vice, more of an exercise in futility and tastelessness.

Oh, to live in an age before you knew everything was bad for you. By the way, if smoking, and drinking, and eating red meat are so bad for you, how come people in the forties looked so great?

This Ain't No Party. This Ain't No Disco— It's AA.

Dear Nuisance Lady,

I think I have a drinking problem. I go out almost every night and have at least, well . . . several drinks. But I don't want to go to AA. The thought of being in some basement room with all those alcoholics talking about their personal problems just makes me cringe. Is it possible to quit drinking without going to AA? There must be another way.

No wAAy

Dear wAAy,

The Nuisance Lady's aunt Lulu felt the same way. Nana Nuisance took her to an AA meeting once, and after it was over she said she'd never needed a drink so much in her life.

Aunt Lulu, now there was a person with a drinking problem. No ifs, ands, or Bacardis about it. She used to walk around from morning till whenever with these big glasses of "lemonade." Even in the winter—when it was two degrees out—she was drinking "lemonade." You wanted to say, "Hey, Aunt Lulu, at least switch to something more seasonal like 'peppermint tea.' "

You could try quitting on your own. Aunt Lulu eventually did. And if *she* could, who can't? But if you do end up going to AA, don't start hanging out with other AAers—roaming the streets in packs, going from coffee shop to coffee shop, speaking the lingo—like the Nuisance Lady's ex-boyfriend Irwin. (It's enough to make you stay a drunk.) Just get your sobering-up support and get out of there.

On the Welcome Wagon

Dear Nuisance Lady,

Is there a proper etiquette about what to say to someone when they come out of rehab? Should it be acknowledged or just ignored? My neighbor, with whom I'm on very friendly terms, is coming home next week and I'm not sure what I should say. Congratulations? That doesn't seem quite right. I'd appreciate any tips, as you seem like the kind of person who has had considerable experience in this area.

DECORUM FOR EX-DRUNKS

Dear Dec,

What do you mean the Nuisance Lady seems like she'd have considerable experience in this area? Listen, lovey, the Nuisance Lady is proud to say that she has never been rehabilitated, not once. She does, however, have many friends and relations who have not been as fortunate—or rather as temperate. According to all the ex-alkies and druggies in the Nuisance Lady's acquaintance, one should not make a big fuss when someone is discharged from a place of enforced abstention, as that only makes the ex-addicted feel self-conscious. A simple *"How's it going, man?"* will do. However, the Nuisance Lady's second cousin, Very Fat Freddy, who tops the record of rehab stays (even he lost count long ago), says, *"I like it when someone gives me a cigar."*

Tanqueray and Turnips

Dear Nuisance Lady,

How can you tell if someone is an alcoholic or not? I'm asking because I think my wife might be one, and I'll tell you why. First, she goes to the bathroom a lot. Second, she hasn't had a bad day in years. Third, she gardens all the time. In the nighttime. In the daytime. In the evening. It doesn't matter. She's constantly cultivating something. What do you think I should do? I've been hesitant to confront her because I have no definite proof. Besides, we get along really well and I don't believe in rocking the boat.

MARRIED TO A LUSH, MAYBE

Dear Lush,

Let me give you a little tip, Sherlock. If she hasn't had a bad day in years, there's no way she's a drunk. Anyone who has ever had any contact, particularly prolonged contact, with a drunk can tell you that they definitely have bad days. Lots of them. Furthermore, compulsive gardening is not necessarily a sign of substance abuse. It could just mean that your wife's a little nuts. Nothing wrong with that. As someone once said, *"Anyone who's not a little crazy is insane."*

As far as the bathroom thing goes, the Nuisance Lady's not a doctor. But if your wife's swigging a lot of water while gardening, you could have your answer. So, unless you start finding bottles of Tanqueray under the turnips, the Nuisance Lady suggests you keep your big mouth shut and just sit back and enjoy your wife's pleasant demeanor. (The men in the Nuisance Lady's family would kill for as much.)

P.S. On second thought, your wife sounds a lot like the Nuisance Lady's great-aunt Gilda, who wore rain hats—all the time—and crocheted compulsively. We just thought she was a little wacky, but after she died we found out she'd been juggling prescriptions for years. Check the medicine cabinet, just to be sure.

Big 'Zac Attack

Dear Nuisance Lady,

I've been feeling depressed for the last few months, so my doctor put me on Prozac. I feel better, but now I can't perform. You see, I'm a performance artist and my work is very morose in a comic sort of way. But since I've been on Prozac, I'm completely uninspired. I've spent hours and hours sitting in my space trying to come up with ideas for new pieces, but . . . nothing. Do you think I should stop taking it? I mean, it does make going grocery shopping easier. But if I can't work who cares about buying broccoli?

No Performance Anxiety

Dear Performance,

The Nuisance Lady ain't too sure about the 'Zac. There's an awful lot of people walking around on 'Zac who should just be walking around and whining a little less. Did you ever see that movie with the short, little British guy who played a drunk guy who married Liza Minnelli? Not that movie. In this one he played a shrink who was treating all these wealthy Park Avenue types, and at the end he had a revelation and told a woman with a poodle, *"You don't have problems, lady. You just have life."*

Besides, a little misery is good material. Hell, it's the only material. Happiness is not funny. If it were, the Nuisance Lady'd be swallowing a six-pack of 'Zac with her morning coffee.

But if you're too depressed to get out of bed or eat any broccoli without the 'Zac, that's a different story. (Hard to get any work done when you're lying on a futon wasting away all day.) Run all this by your doctor—the Nuisance Lady hasn't been one since that incident with Stevie Sandler in the second grade—and read Virginia Woolf. She's always good for some creative-woman-in-a-cubicle inspiration.

No, You're Not a Soul Man

Dear Nuisance Lady,

I just found a joint under a Zeppelin CD and I'm so mad I could spit. I know it's my husband's. He promised me he wouldn't smoke pot anymore. It's not that I mind him smoking a joint once in a while; I don't.

The problem is that we've been trying to conceive a baby for the last year and a half and so far—nothing. When we went to a doctor, we found out that my husband has a low sperm count. Well, guess what makes a man's sperm count low? Marijuana, that's what. He promised me he would stop smoking until after we conceived, but he hasn't obviously. Don't you think he's being totally selfish?

MARRIED TO CHEECH, OR CHONG

Dear Chong,

All the Nuisance Lady can say is, if that were her husband, that joint is the only thing his lips would be touching. Selfish doesn't begin to cover it. First of all, he shouldn't be smoking pot when you're trying to get pregnant. Period. It could affect the child. The poor little thing could be born with a guitar in its hand, strumming chords of "Sweet Home Alabama" or "Hotel California." What if it's a boy? And God help you if you're white. The only thing worse than a white boy with a guitar is a white boy with a guitar and a fireplace. Last New Year's the Nuisance Lady's Free-Birding friend Sam was so bad that someone—from across the room—"accidentally" burned two of his guitar strings off with their Zippo lighter.

Anyway, the Nuisance Lady wouldn't even consider having a child with such a man. He's obviously not ready for fatherhood. For God's sake, if John Lennon could stop smoking pot long enough to get Yoko knocked up . . .

I Swear, Mom, It Was Something I Ate

Dear Nuisance Lady,

My son came home drunk last night. He tried to hide it, but I knew. He tripped on the linoleum four times. (I haven't waxed the floor in days.) And he poured three glasses of milk and then didn't drink them. I haven't said anything to him yet, because he's still sleeping it off. I'm not sure how to handle this. Should I take away his privileges? Should tell him he has to get counseling? Should I ground him until graduation?

VERY BEERY BOY

Dear Beery,

Hopefully, the kid has better judgment than you, honey. Ground him—for a week. Take away one of his privileges— the beer-drinking one. But don't overreact. Every kid comes home drunk a couple of times in high school, but it does not, contrary to what commercials with eggs and really bad actors playing crack dealers would have you believe, necessarily mean he'll end up a junkie-whore who lives on the street, holds up liquor stores, spends some time in jail, and talks to his shoes.

If the kid's snorting smack every day before study hall, then you've got something to worry about. Or if he sniffs glue— even once. Because that would indicate that he ain't all that bright to begin with, and can't afford to lose even a single brain cell.

P.S. If you really want to get him, don't say anything. That's what Mama Nuisance did the first time the Nuisance Lady came home a little liquored up. It's sheer torture. You just sit there . . . waiting. Waiting for the big Mama shoe to drop and kick you in the ass.

Drinking and Dialing Don't Mix

Dear Nuisance Lady,

You know those mornings when you wake up and, for a few sweet, sweet seconds, it's all just a blank. But then it comes back. Like a punch in the gut. That's me and that's this morning. I'm never ever drinking again. Even if someone put a gun to my head and said drink this glass of Cabarnet or die, I wouldn't do it.

I went out with my girlfriends last night. They were trying to cheer me up because this guy I'd been seeing, and was really starting to like, dumped me for some chick named Virginia from Virginia who works for ESPN.

Well, to make a long and still oh-so-painful story short, I called him from a bar at 2:30 in the morning and begged him to take me back. I actually cried and slurred *"but we can work it out"* a million times.

It gets worse. When he finally hung up on me, I called back again and again. Then, when he wouldn't pick up the phone anymore, I went over to his apartment and rang his buzzer again and again, until some passing stranger took pity on me and put me in a cab. I want to die. I want someone to kill me. Will you kill me, Nuisance Lady?

TOO DRUNK AND STUPID TO LIVE

Dear Drunk and Stupid,

Sorry to disappoint you, sweets, but there're a lot of people the Nuisance Lady'd kill before she'd kill you: ex-boyfriends, ex-bosses, and lots of family members.

Anyway, what we've got here is another statistic, another sad case of DWI: Dialing While Intoxicated. And in your case, there was even a little D and B involved: Drinking and Buzzing. (Luckily for you, he didn't answer and a face-to-face confrontation was narrowly avoided.)

Everybody's been there, sister. Once, when the Nuisance Lady was suffering from a bad case of Dewar's and why-are-all-these-other-broads-walking-around-with-my-husband(s)?, she called her sophomore-year boyfriend in Seattle at six in the morning to vigorously demand the return of her Dead Kennedys' tape and her people-in-Kuala-Lumpur-are-walking-around-in-them Black Dog T-shirt. She woke up his wife, his newborn, his nephews, and his entire computer-literate, nature-loving neighborhood. Don't worry. In five or six years it'll no longer seem unbearable, only appalling.

P.S. Don't drink and dial. Next time hide the phone; break your own fingers if you have to. And where were your friends? Friends don't let friends dial drunk. They should have taken your quarters.

Wedded: Bliss or Miss

*C*ompromise is the key to a good marriage. But how long can you keep that up for? So when you stop compromising, you'd better start bickering. Bicker, bicker, bicker. The more bickering the better; because when you live with the same person night and day, day and night, and even on weekends, they're bound—with a big B—to start driving you crazy eventually. And much better to be a bickering couple than a no-talking couple. (The no talking'll kill you every time or at least make you wish something would kill you.) In fact, there's not much difference between bickering and doing the cha-cha. You're on the dance floor of life, you've got your partner (unless some little twenty-two-year-old slut cuts in), and you're feeling good. You start out with a little cheek-to-cheek, but then somebody steps on somebody's feet, and before you know it you're doing the cha-cha: "We can't afford a new car." *Cha-cha-cha.* "We could if you gave up your golf lessons." *Cha-cha-cha.* But the cha-cha's a hell of a lot better than the hustle, at least you're still touching. Do the hustle, don, don, don, don, are divorce lawyers listed under D or L?

■

And You Thought Three Carats Was Too Much

Dear Nuisance Lady,

I'm in love with a jeweler. Most women would probably consider this a plus. Especially since his sister just told me that he's designing a special engagement ring for me: a flawless three-carat diamond encircled by two rows of rubies in an antique platinum setting. I know this might sound ungrateful, but I really don't want it. In fact, I don't want a ring at all. What I really want is a horse. I've always dreamed of owning my own horse, but haven't quite been able to afford it. Do you think it would be too rude of me to tell my boyfriend that I'd rather have a horse as an engagement present?

NO RING, PLEASE

Dear No Ring,

Have you lost your mind? An engagement horse? (What are you going to do, walk around with a string on your finger attached to a horse? *"Oh, have you seen my engagement horse?"*) The song, toots, does not go, *"Palominos are a girl's best friend."* Accept the ring, ecstatically, and work the poor schnook over for a horse on the honeymoon.

Death of a Housewife: No More Meat Loaf

Dear Nuisance Lady,

Perhaps you could help me. My wife wants to get pregnant. And I don't want her to. It's not that I don't want kids. I do—

someday. But we've only been married a year and I'm not making that much money, not enough for her to stay home after the baby's born, which is what she wants. I just don't understand why she has to have a baby right now. She's only twenty-eight, so there's no rush. We've got a lot of time to have children. Every time we try to discuss it, she ends up crying and I come off like a bad guy. Do you think I should just give in and agree to start a family?

NOT READY YET

Dear Yet,

Question: Does your wife like her job? If the answer is no, she might be suffering from *overeducated-career-frustrated-middle-class-chick-got-to-get-myself-knocked-up-but-quick* syndrome, which, by the way, cannot be made into a cutesy acronym. The Nuisance Lady, brilliant social observer that she is, has noticed that this syndrome is very prevalent among chicks in their late twenties, early thirties. That, of course, being the time when people suddenly wake up one morning and realize that their careers either aren't going as well as they had hoped or that they don't have one at all. Now, men, because of biological limitations and social conventions, have no choice but to either scramble like hell to find themselves a more meaningful *métier* or else resign themselves to a Willy Lomanesque existence.

But women have a third option: *baby*. (Mere marriage is not enough anymore, since society finds women without children who stay at home utterly unacceptable. Gone are the ladies of leisure, sitting home, watching a few soaps, eating a few bonbons, taking a few sips of sherry, making an occasional meat loaf. Damn, there was a very short window of opportunity in between the invention of modern conveniences and the advent of the career woman, and the Nuisance Lady missed it.)

Anyway, if your wife fits this profile, you might want to have a serious and dry-eyed discussion with her about her career—finding a new one, getting one, whatever it takes. But—DO NOT have children until both of you are financially and emotionally ready. If you let her pressure you into having kids now, you'll end up resenting it sooner or later, and that's no good for a marriage.

Men Seeking Men (with Salt-and-Pepper Mustaches)

Dear Nuisance Lady,

My sister is married to a musician/record producer. (We'll call him Marzipan.) Several months ago my sister noticed strange numbers on the phone bill, which turned out to be assorted MEN SEEKING MEN sex lines.

To make an extremely long and tearful story short, Marzipan admitted that he had made the calls, and that he has a thing for older men with salt-and-pepper mustaches. (His father died when he was nine.) Then he informed my sister that he was moving to Japan to study some kind of ancient Japanese drum beating.

I know this sounds like the plot of a silly sitcom, but the really sad side of it is that my sister hasn't gotten out of bed in weeks. I want to help, but I don't know what to do for her. Do you have any ideas?

ONE SAD SISTER

■   ■   ■

Dear Sister,

The Nuisance Lady must take this opportunity to say something to all the men in our fair land: IF YOU'RE GAY, DON'T, DON'T MARRY A WOMAN.

Seems fairly logical to some, but evidently not to others. The Nuisance Lady well remembers the look on the face of her favorite social studies teacher—Mrs. Warren—the day she came back to school after finding her husband—Mr. Warren—in bed with his broker.

Now, as to your sister: Before the next strip of sunlight seeps over the Statue of Liberty's sarong she should be sitting front and center at a support-group meeting. And tell her to hang in there—just like that little kitten doing a chin-up on that oh-so-ubiquitous seventies poster. Things'll get better. By the time the Nuisance Lady had graduated from high school, Mrs. Warren had started to smile again and was dating Mr. Mozecki, the algebra teacher.

P.S. That Japanese drum-beating thing is called *taiko*, and it is in fact an ancient art that requires a lifetime of study.

Too Hard to Handle

Dear Nuisance Lady,

I was wondering if you could help me with my wife. Last year she decided she wanted to get into shape, which was a good thing. But now she's gone overboard. She spends four to five hours a day in the gym, drinks all kinds of weird metabolic protein shakes, and, quite frankly, is beginning to look like one of my son's Morphin Power Rangers in drag. I find this extremely unattractive. Call me old-fashioned, but I like to see a few curves, touch something that isn't as hard as a butcher-block table. What can I do, Nuisance Lady? I don't want to start a fight or hurt my wife's feelings, but I really want her to stop all this before it's too late.

IT'S TOO HARD

Dear Hard,

What's that you say? Your wife's body is too hard. Life is too hard. You should try being a broad, buddy. Here's a sample of what it's like: *Don't eat. Don't eat. Don't eat. Work out. Use weights. Don't gain weight. Eat pasta. Don't eat pasta. Breasts not big enough. No movie theater popcorn. Hey, where are the breasts? Put that piece of bread down. Butt's too big. No butter, please. No salad dressing, either. Size 6? Well, not exactly. Hips! Try power walking.*

So, as you can tell, a lot of sympathy for you the Nuisance Lady ain't got. But why not suggest to your wife that instead of going to the gym you go out for a big romantic lunch, or stay home and eat Oreo-mint ice cream and smoked oysters in bed?

OK, He's Not Exactly Rin-Tin-Tin

Dear Nuisance Lady,

My wife and I've decided to get each other a dog for our anniversary, one dog between the two of us. But my wife, for some completely weird reason, wants to get a small dog, you know, the kind that wear bows in their hair. I said no way am I walking down the street with some little frou-frou in pink. I want a real dog, a man's dog—a Lab or a shepherd. Everyone is going to think I'm a gay man for God's sake. But she won't budge. She says it's the Chihuahua or nothing. Isn't she being unreasonable, Nuisance Lady? Please tell her she's being unreasonable.

DOG GONNED

Dear Dog,

All right, pal. First of all, you've already got the one accessory that usually (but not always) precludes homosexuality—a wife. So your friends and relations probably already know you're not a gay man. And who the hell cares what people walking down the street think? (Most of them could use a small dog to draw attention away from themselves.)

As to the actual pooch, everyone knows that not only real men but also real women prefer real dogs: dogs that don't fit in a bread basket or wear bows; dogs that can't be used in lieu of a soccer ball in a jam.

How about a nice spaniel? Springer, perhaps? That's a good compromise—not too big, not too little. Classy-looking but doesn't wear unnecessary accessories. (Unless you put one of those stupid sweaters on him. Hello, the dog's already wearing one, knit by Mother Nature.) Anyway, just remember compromise is the key to a healthy, manageable marriage. Right.

P.S. The French have a saying: *"All I ask is to be reincarnated as a rich man's mistress or a gay man's dog."* (Personally, the Nuisance Lady'd prefer to come back as the scruffy.)

You Can't Expect a Hot Lunch Every Day

Dear Nuisance Lady,

My wife just isn't attractive to me anymore. I don't know what to do. I don't want to be one of those guys who fool around. But I look at my wife and . . . nothing. I mean I still love her and respect her, but sexually, nothing. I don't know why I feel like this. It's not as though she's gotten fat or anything. She looks pretty much the same as she did when we got married. What do I do? As I said, I don't want to fool around, but lately I've been noticing other women more and more.

BOB

Dear Bob,

"My wife just isn't attractive to me anymore." The Nuisance Lady wishes she had one of those big boxing gloves with the cranks. One with an incredibly long reach, so she could just crank it and it would reach right across Manhattan into your office and bang you on the head. Listen, Rico Suave, the Nuisance Lady would give you ten to one that your wife's not looking at you and screaming, *"Whoa, hot lunch on toast."*

It's obvious that you and your wife are experiencing a slight lull in the sea of conjugal passion. So, might the Nuisance Lady suggest marital aids? You know, maybe one of those kits where one or both of you dress up like corseted damsels-in-distress. Just a suggestion. But seriously, swing from the chandeliers, light yourselves up like Christmas trees. Do whatever it takes. And if absolutely nothing works, sit tight, fantasize a little, and just ride it out because, inevitably, one morning you will wake up, look over at your wife and think, *"Aay, Chihuahua."*

P.S. Just remember Bob, it's easy, especially for a man, to find someone whose boots you want to knock. But it ain't nearly as easy to find someone you love and respect.

One Rabbi to Go, Please

Dear Nuisance Lady,

Can I tell you about something that is killing me? I mean, I'm literally dying. I can hear my heart stopping even as I write this letter. My son is getting married this summer to a shiksa. (That's a girl who's not Jewish, in case you didn't know.) I'm not happy about this. How could I be happy? But I accept. What can I do? But now he tells me that the ceremony is being performed by a justice of the peace. No rabbi. This I can't accept. I know it's possible to have a rabbi even if you're marrying a goy, because my friend Frieda's son, who also married a shiksa, had a rabbi and a reverend at his wedding. I mentioned this to my son—the one with no respect for his mother's feelings—but he says it's already been decided.

SUFFERING IN SILENCE

Dear Suffering,

You may be suffering, but you ain't doing it in silence, honey. The Nuisance Lady can hear your guilt-inducing sighs and "silent" weeping from here. That's okay. The more guilt the better. Guilt'll get you everywhere, at least where your children are concerned. The Nuisance Lady knows this. She has the mother to prove it. Just tell your son how much it would mean to you to have a rabbi perform at least part of the ceremony. Tell him how you've dreamed of this day ever since he was a little boy. Remind him that you're not getting any younger. Then for the *pièce de résistance say, "Just remember that whatever you decide I'm your mother and I'll love you and support you no matter what."* Ten bucks says that'll get you a rabbi front and center.

Well Groomed

Dear Nuisance Lady,

Last weekend I went to a really chi chi engagement party. I was having a great time—dancing, drinking, eating little shrimp wrapped in paper—until the future groom made a pass at me. At first, I wasn't sure. I thought maybe I was just mistaking friendliness for flirtiness. But when he cornered me on my way to the bathroom and asked me to "feel his muscle," I knew that I could no longer give him the benefit of the doubt.

Do you think I should tell his fiancée? I really feel she has the right to know that she's marrying the dirtiest of dogs. On the other hand, the little piggy's sister is one of my best friends, and I don't want to get embroiled in a whole family thing.

THE OBJECT OF ENGAGED AFFECTIONS

Dear Object,

Honey, honey, honey. Never tell anybody anything. The Nuisance Lady knows. She's had grooms hanging all over her like cheap suits. In fact, one amorous idiot even proposed a little yakahoola in the vestry, vestuary, whatever, just seconds after promising to forsake all others. To hell with "as long as they both shall live"; until after the reception ended would have been nice.

Anyway, keep your mouth shut. And, if it happens again, just tell him that you're not interested in feeling any of his muscles, wherever they may be. (In the Nuisance Lady's vast experience, one or two "back off, big broncos" is enough for most men.) Have a great time at the wedding, if it ever takes place, and talk to single guys at the reception.

Also, in the future, please remember what the Nuisance Lady's sporadically sage, middle-aged aunt Catty always says, *"Men are never friendly to women between the ages of fifteen and fifty-five."*

Dearly Nearly Naked Beloved

Dear Nuisance Lady,

My best friend says you shouldn't wear a sexy dress to a wedding. He says it's inappropriate. He had a fit when he saw the little black dress I was planning to wear to his brother's wedding. I say I can wear whatever I want, since I'm doing him a favor by going with him after his girlfriend dumped him at the last minute. After all, I'll have to put up with his letchy cousin Robby chasing me around all night.

WONDERING ABOUT WEDDING ATTIRE

■   ■   ■

Dear WAWA,

Always follow this simple rule: *If it covers both cheeks and nipples with a little more than a couple of inches to spare, then it's okay.* If your friend continues to find fault with your frock, then just say what the Nuisance Lady did when her friend Carl made a fuss about the slinky shift she wore to his boss's wedding, *"Excuuuuse me for not wearing some Kelly green frump job from Talbots like the rest of the corporate clones' spouses. I'm going to the buffet table."*

And the Bride Wore...Diapers

Dear Nuisance Lady,

My son came home last night and told us he was getting married. My wife and I were stunned. It's not that we don't like the girl. She's a lovely girl from a good family. However, our son is only twenty-four and has just graduated from law school. My wife and I think he should wait to get married until he's established himself in his profession and perhaps dated a few more girls. Jenny, his fiancée, is really his first serious girlfriend. I want to talk to him about this, but my wife says he'll only resent it and we'll end up starting off on the wrong foot with Jenny.

TOO SOON

Dear TS,

Relax, buddy, your son is no mere anomaly. He's part of a trend. Last weekend the Nuisance Lady went to a wedding where the bride must've been twelve.

Society is just one giant pendulum that keeps swinging back and forth, back and forth. Right now it's swinging toward getting engaged in junior high. Maybe it's because of AIDS, maybe it's because these kids grew up in the Reagan era (although you'd think seeing Ron and Nancy would've pushed them the other way). Maybe it's because all their parents are divorced ten times over. Or because these young broads are looking at the Nuisance Lady and her single friends and saying to themselves, *"That ain't going to be me."*

Anyway, for whatever reason, it's like we're in the Appalachians all of a sudden. Don't worry. In the long run they aren't going to end up any better or worse than people who waited to get married. We're all just hanging on to the pendulum, swinging back and forth.

Bitches in White

Dear Nuisance Lady,

I think my fiancée has lost her mind. First, she made me and my groomsmen buy (no rentals for her, not good enough) tuxedos that cost more money than . . . well, an indecent amount of money. Then she made my sister spend an even more ridiculous amount on a bridesmaid's dress. Then she insisted that I get first-class tickets for our honeymoon. (Coach was out of the question.) Then she decided the champagne we were going to serve wasn't good enough. We had to upgrade. Oh, and I almost forgot about the lobster. She's got to serve lobster. Lobster for 150 people. I thought I was marrying a nice, sweet, sensible girl, but now I'm not so sure. I swear I'm almost having second thoughts. Is this what life with her is going to be like?

ABOUT TO BE WED WORRIED GUY

Dear Wed Guy,

Fear not, intended one, brides-to-be get hormones that course through their nervous systems at 190 miles an hour. These hormones turn them into *bibis*—bridal bitches. Smart women, sensible women, neurosurgeons, federal judges suddenly spend hours agonizing over *braised radicchio and goat cheese wrapped in phyllo dough* versus *artichoke and porcini mushroom–filled empanadas*. The Nuisance Lady knew one *bibi* who insisted upon having the room where her reception was being held rewallpapered because the existing wallpaper didn't match the bridesmaids' dresses. Another excessively eager *bibi* even requested that the Nuisance Lady bind her breasts with special breastbinding tape because said *bibi* didn't want any chesty bridesmaids spoiling the lines of the luscious lemon chiffon gowns she had selected. So, if you're smart you'll do as all good grooms do—smile and answer, *"Whatever you say, honey."* And don't worry, as soon as the whole thing is over, your fiancée will once again become the same lovely, sane woman you fell in love with.

It Don't Mean a Thing
If You Ain't Got That Ring

Dear Nuisance Lady,

Six months ago I moved to a new city so I could be with my boyfriend, Dennis. After five years of back and forth, we decided it was time. Of course, I was expecting to get engaged upon my arrival or shortly thereafter. But so far there's been nothing, not even the vaguest hint of a velvet box. (I've been checking his jacket pockets and dresser drawers regularly.) What do you think this means? Should I give him an ultimatum or wait patiently a little longer?

Breathlessly Awaiting Betrothal

Dear Babs,

The Nuisance Lady thinks this means that if you've already bought the dress, which she'll bet you did, you should take it back—or cut it into something cocktail length.

Have you ever heard of Trent's Two-Year Rule, named after the wise old lobsterman who made it? (Actually, he's a hip, mod, Generation X–type lobsterman. What else could he be with a name like Trent?) Trent's Two-Year Rule, simply put, is that if you aren't bound or at least betrothed within two years, you aren't going to be. The theory being that something's blocking it, usually one or both bodies secretly searching for somebody else.

So, little Godot, the Nuisance Lady suggests you do what Trent does when he gets a tough lobster—throw it back in the ocean and keep on fishing.

P.S. Ten-to-one if you walk out on him, he'll be completely shocked and won't understand why. The Nuisance Lady recently received a 4:00 A.M. phone call from her friend Rick the Rocker. His girlfriend, Bettina the Ballerina, had just walked out on him. He was completely overwrought, taken aback. *"Hello, you've been going out with her for six years, living together for five of them, and she finally left you because you won't marry her. The part of this you don't understand . . . would be?"*

It's an Antique

Dear Nuisance Lady,

Do you know what I'm spending the whole summer doing? Going to weddings. I have a wedding to go to every single weekend from Memorial Day to Labor Day. Some weekends I have two or three. I know I've got to go to some of them— my sister's, my college roommate's, etc. But some invitations are just ridiculous. Last week I got one in the mail, and it took me three days to figure out how I knew them. Come on. Do I have to get these meet-them-once-at-a-party-and-they-invite-you-to-their-wedding types a gift? After all, even a cheap gift is expensive these days.

TOO MANY WEDDINGS, TOO LITTLE SUMMER

Dear Weddings,

Please, honey, you should be glad you're not a McJew. Weddings are hell. Between the drinking with the Irish half of the family and the eating with the Jewish half, you're sick for days after. And if the Latin in-laws show up, there's dancing. Then you're sick before you get home.

And the cousins. They're all nuts. Like Cousin Dorie. She thinks she was a member of the 1958 equestrian team. She wasn't born until '62 and has never been near a horse in her life. It's so hard to believe they can find people to marry them.

Anyway, of course, you don't have to get gifts for these don't-have-enough-real-friends-to-fill-a-banquet-hall types. If you ever run into one of them somewhere, just say, *"Oh, I hope you liked the antique egg-chopper I sent."* They'll never know the difference, and they'll feel guilty about not sending a thank-you note.

The Three Fs—
Friendship, Fighting,
and Fashion

Never, never, never, ever tell anybody anything. The less people know—how much money you make, who you've slept with—the less they have to hold against you. The Nuisance Lady learned this at the knee of Great-Grandma Nuisance. And it wasn't until her funeral that everyone found out she was rich as bejeezuz and had slept with all her friends' husbands. By then, what did she care?

▪

Reality, Like Your Bustline, Can Be Easily Enhanced

Dear Nuisance Lady,

I have a friend who's, who's . . . prone to exaggeration. Everything she does becomes this incredible feat. Like she started going to the gym and now she's "training for the Ironman." I want to say, "Hello, twenty minutes on the Lifecycle is not training for the Ironman." Last week she made Pillsbury Doughboy chocolate-chip cookies, and now she's opening her own Viennese pastry shop.

It's gotten so bad that every time I go out with her I just shake my head, "uh, uh, uh." But I really want to leap across the table, backhand her a couple of times, and scream, "LIAR. LIAR. LIAR." Then again, she's a really good friend whom I've known forever. Should I call her on this stuff or just continue to ignore her? Or dump her as a friend?

EXASPERATED

Dear Exasperated,

Honey, honey, honey. Don't be so hard on your friend. She's just a solipsist. Solipsists believe that reality is like Play-Doh: You can mold it to whatever shape you want.

In the Nuisance Lady's family there are more solipsists than you can shake a stick at—we're devout. Take Grandpa Nuisance. A poor, old, almost blind woman once mistook him for Errol Flynn at a Schrafft's counter. But good little solipsist that he is, this really meant that movie studios—MGM, Warner Brothers, all the greats—were banging on his door begging him to sign contracts. (He chose to become an insurance broker instead. Go figure.)

And Grandma Nuisance—one other poor schlub besides Grandpa Nuisance asked her to marry him. Hundreds, thousands of men were down on their hands and knees begging her to marry them. They were on top of the Empire State Building threatening to throw themselves off if she didn't marry them. Rich men. Handsome men. Famous men. Rich, handsome, and famous. (But, of course, she picked the insurance broker who looked just like Errol Flynn.)

So, have some respect for your friend's devotions and try to appreciate the fact that at least she's not boring. A healthy dose of solipsism isn't such a bad thing, and it goes well with a little strudel.

All Dressed Up and No Place to Flaunt

Dear Nuisance Lady,

I know you must hear really stupid ideas all the time, but I have to tell you about the most idiotic one of all time. My best friend is having a surprise birthday party for my other best friend and—get this—it's an all-girl, black-tie party. I ask you, have you ever heard of anything more nonsensical in your entire life?

TUXEDO

P.S. She says she wants it to be an "elegant evening."

Dear Tuxedo,

Are you and your friends lesbians? If not, then the Nuisance Lady tends to agree with you. It's not that she doesn't see the benefit of a chicks' night. She can and she does. But personally speaking, if the Nuisance Lady's going to get all gussied up—heels, little black dress, the whole deal—she wants to get some smoldering glances and long, lustful looks with a few cleavage peeks thrown in. She also wants the chance to do some eyelash batting, hair flipping, and intimate lean-ins. Otherwise, just throw on an old pair of Levi's and you're good to go. That's just the Nuisance Lady, though.

P.S. The Nuisance Lady asked if you guys were lesbians because if you are, then an all-girl party would obviously have an entirely different meaning and make much more sense.

Fantasyland Is Right Next to Never-Never Land

Dear Nuisance Lady,

Recently, a very good friend of mine told me that he frequently fantasized about me. I was SHOCKED. Of course, I couldn't help asking him exactly what his fantasies were, and exactly what I was wearing in them. He completely clammed up, claimed that it was "personal" and "private."

Excuse me, but if I'm starring in these smutty scenarios, then I think I have a right to know what it is I'm doing, don't you? Furthermore, I think this will affect our friendship, because now every time we're together, I'll wonder if he's picturing me in peekaboo panties.

FANTASIA

Dear Fantasia,

Sweets, I'm going to tell you something that every woman over the age of ten with two brain cells to rub together knows: MEN FANTASIZE ABOUT EVERYONE ALL THE TIME. That's what makes them men.

However, when a man confesses this to a particular pal, it usually means he would like to cross the frontier from fantasyland into adventureland. If you're not interested in any capers with your comrade, just say what the Nuisance Lady did when her friend Spencer told her that he regularly "thought" about her at the tanning parlor: *"I think I'll have the kung pao shrimp."*

Walking Talk Shows

Dear Nuisance Lady,

What can you do about people who don't stop talking? There is this woman in my office who is always telling me her personal problems. I know about her nephew's divorce from "that trashy, tacky little thing," her sister-in-law's affair with the Lebanese shoe designer, her husband's problems with his boss, her son's problems at school, her neighbor's alcoholic daughter, and every one of her daughter's diets, in detail. I've had it. How do I politely tell this woman that I'm not interested in her private life?

DELUGED WITH DRIVEL

Dear Drivel,

Your letter brings back not-so-fond memories of the eighties and coke-induced confessions like, *"When I was fifteen I had sex with my half sister"* from some jaw-snapping fool you'd just met at the bar five minutes ago. Eh, in the eighties they had coke, in the nineties they have talk shows. Same thing.

Anyway, it's impossible to be tactful with these people. They have no understanding of what is and is not appropriate. If they did, they wouldn't be standing in front of the water cooler telling you about how their husbands are having trouble maintaining erections lately. Next time Babbling Betty starts going on, just say, *"Excuse me, does this directly involve me in any way? No? Well then, I'd rather not hear about it."*

P.S. If that doesn't work, you can always do what Mrs. Felzenhower at the Nuisance Lady's old office did whenever she was approached by anyone—even people asking legitimate, work-related questions: Begin typing furiously and mutter, *"Get away from me. Get away from me. Get away from me."*

Ass-thetically Speaking

Dear Nuisance Lady,

My friend Jim used to be the greatest guy. The kind you could hang out with, shoot hoops with . . . But ever since he got this job at a highbrow publishing house, he's been unbearable. He's constantly making these ridiculous literary references—like the other day he said that my new Nikes were very Nabokovian (I'm not kidding). Then he said my bulldog, Sally, reminded him of Eustacia Vye in *The Return of the Native*. Is that the stupidest thing you've ever heard? I really like Jim, but I just can't take him for one more second. Should I tell him that he's become a pompous pain in my ass?

ABSOLUTELY NOT NABOKOVIAN

P.S. Oh, by the way, I'm not supposed to call him Jim anymore. It's James now. I feel like telling him that James was the friggin chauffeur's name: *"Home, James. Home."*

Dear Nab,

Pretensions, there's nothing worse than people who get pretensions—literary ones, linguistic ones, culinary ones. They start saying the word "aesthetic" and it's all down hill from there: *"You want french fries or a baked potato with that?" "Well, aesthetically . . ."* You want to go to the Laundromat with me?" "*The aesthetics of the situation . . ."*

You should've seen the Nuisance Lady's friend Kim when she got a job working at a hoity-toity auction house. She changed her look with every sale. They auctioned off the Dutch masters—Van Eyck, Vermeer, and so on. She got one of those little Dutch boy haircuts, like the kid on the paint can, and walked around in a pair of three-hundred-dollar clogs. Then, when they were selling stuff from the Ming dynasty, she stuffed herself into a Suzy Wong dress and asked people to call her Kimono: "Will not."

You could tell your friend he's become a pretentious little twit, but he won't listen. People never believe anything about themselves they don't want to: *"So what if I had ten Myers's and OJ at brunch? Doesn't mean I have a drinking problem."*

Just ride it out. He'll settle down, eventually. Kim got fired from the auction house and now works as a receptionist at her local congressman's office. You should see the outfits she's wearing now. (The gun-control slip dress really was a bit much—all that fake blood.)

Buddha Pests

Dear Nuisance Lady,

My husband and I recently purchased a lovely home in the country. We've been spending as much time there as my husband's business commitments permit and would have had an utterly glorious summer except for one small fly in the ointment—our neighbors. They are practicing Buddhists, quite practicing. They're out on their lawn every morning at six o'clock sharp—chanting. One would have thought that Buddhist chanting has a mellifluous, almost entrancing sound. It does not. It sounds, as my husband puts it, "like somebody's trying to skin a big old tomcat."

They also have group sessions where other Buddhists come and play music, chant some more, and read aloud, loudly, from the works of the Dalai Lama. My husband and I are at a loss. We don't want to stop anyone from exercising their constitutional right to practice their religion. However, we do feel that we are entitled to a little tranquility in our own home. What is your opinion?

BOTHERED BY BUDDHISTS

Dear Triple B,

Nobody's allowed to do anything if it's too loud. That is the Nuisance Lady's opinion. And something the three Venezuelan disco kings next door fail to understand: *"At the Copa, Copa Cabana. The hottest spot north of Havana . . . There was blood and a single gunshot, but just who shot who?"* (Hey, Rico shot Tony. That's who shot who. And he's coming for you next if you don't turn that down.)

But, Buddhists—you don't usually hear about them causing too much trouble. They seem like a nice bunch, except for that weenie Richard Gere. Anyway, lovey, you march yourself right over to that Buddhist temple next door and say, *"Lovely that you find your religious practices so gratifying, soul-nourishing and all that, but please keep it down."* If that doesn't work, try hurling chunks of meat over the hedges. I hear they're all vegetarians.

Is There a Priest in the House?

Dear Nuisance Lady,

This summer I took a share in a beach house with people I met through a friend. The house is nice and everyone gets along really well, except for one small problem: There's a priest in the house. Literally. Since I'm from your typical quasi-observant Irish Catholic family, his presence makes me feel uncomfortable doing the things one normally does in a summer house: drinking, having sex, wearing small amounts of clothing. I don't know what to do. I'm tempted to ask for my money back. But I don't want to start a fight or hurt Father————'s feelings. He's very nice. I also want someplace to go on the weekends.

UNCOMFORTABLE CATHOLIC

Dear Catholic,

Why, for the love of Saint Somebody, isn't the priest in a priest place? The Nuisance Lady hasn't been practicing lately— at least not anything religious—so she isn't up on the latest ecclesiastical etiquette. But shouldn't priests be out performing weddings or teaching all the little Catholic kids who failed something and have to go to summer school?

Well, one can only assume that a priest who takes a summer share must be open-minded, and won't try to turn your weekends into retreats. Also, remember that you're an adult and entitled to live your life as you wish. A priest, or any other person of the cloth, is there to offer help and comfort to those who seek it, not to judge those who do not.

Consider the advantages: on-site confession after a night of sinning and someone who actually knows all Ten Commandments, should the subject ever come up.

P.S. What are priests wearing on the beach these days?

Prescribe 'Em, Drugstore Cowboy

Dear Nuisance Lady,

My roommate is a big wacko. Ever since I've known him he's had something: knee problems, back problems, regularity problems. Our apartment is overflowing with braces, crutches, canes, heating pads, ice packs. You should see the medicine chest: Videx, Zovirax, Zithromax . . . Once in college, he had to take four final exams with malaria. Malaria. He hadn't been south of Jersey since he was fourteen. But he had malaria.

To top it all off, we've now been banned from both our neighborhood pharmacies. The other day we were standing at the counter waiting to get one of his prescriptions filled, when the lady in front of us starts describing her allergy symptoms and asking the pharmacist what she should take. I can see my roommate starting to sweat and shake. "Claritin, he's got to say Claritin," he keeps muttering to himself. I told him to calm down, but he kept saying, "But, it's an obvious call, man, it's Claritin. Claritin." I had to drag him out of there as he was yelling, "And you call yourself a pharmacist?" Help me, Nuisance Lady. Is there anything that can be done?

ROOMMATE WITHOUT A REMEDY

■   ■   ■

Dear Roommate,

No. Hypochondriacs or the "medically aware," as they like to be called, have a chronic condition. Take the Nuisance Lady's aunt Phyllis who went to the doctor's more than to D'Agostino's—and she went to D'Agostino's a lot. The woman died at ninety-seven after outliving eleven doctors and surviving thousands of "fatal illnesses." She had query fever—a disease common in areas where sheep and goats are herded—at least three times. She lived in Brooklyn. The good thing about it was that every time you went to her house she gave you some of her stuff, "a little remembrance," since that would probably be "the last time" you ever saw her. Free stuff. Try asking your roommate for his stereo or skis. Also, make him deal only with pharmacies that deliver. Other than that, there's nothing you can do. It's a thing and everybody's got them.

Hey, Mr. Stork, Just Drop the Baby Off and Go

Dear Nuisance Lady,

My neighbors and I are about to have a doozey of a fight. They had a baby a couple of months ago. Well, the morning after the baby is born, I walk outside of my house to get the paper and what do I see? A horror, that's what I see. I see this six-foot stork with a giant cigar in his mouth and a big pink banner that says, *Maria Theresa* ————. *Born November 12, 1995. 7.6 lbs., etc., etc.*

Who ever heard of such a thing? Even though it killed me, I

said to myself, "Okay, Rita, don't say anything. Why make trouble? It'll be gone in a few days." That was two months and eighteen days ago. The kid's already crawling, for God's sake. It'll be graduating from high school and they'll still have that thing out there. Or maybe they'll wait until they have the second kid and just cross out the name. I've tried to graciously suggest that it's time for the stork to fly south, but they ignore me. What should I do?

SICK OF THE STORK

Dear Stork,

The Nuisance Lady would've known the neighbors were Italian, even if you hadn't said the kid's name. Definitely the only ethnic group that would go for the stork. Hey, Hispanics, maybe. Anyway, you've been patient long enough. It's time to kill the stork. Make a midnight raid. Drop the bird at the dump. If questioned by your neighbors or the local police, blame it on the neighborhood kids, those tricksters. Shake your head sympathetically and say, *"They were probably on drugs. They're all on drugs, you know."* May the gods of tasteful lawn decorations be with you. And if they've got any Christmas decorations still up, take those too. No Nativity scenes after New Year's. When will people learn?

Buy Me a River

Dear Nuisance Lady,

I'm really worried about my roommate. His girlfriend dumped him for another guy. They'd been going out for four years and he was really crazy about her. (Personally, I didn't think she was all that great.)

Ever since she dumped him, all he's done is buy stuff—skis, cross-country ski machines, cordless power drills, camcorders, police sirens, ladders, laptops, lots of stuff with polar fleece, track lights, Eddy Merckx racing bikes, electric toothbrushes, tiny telephones, automated martini shakers, massaging mattresses, tons of sh– from Sharper Image.

Yesterday, I came home and there was a friggin' kayak in the middle of the living room. I tripped over it this morning on my way to the new espresso machine. I'm trying to be sympathetic, but give me a break. And some more space.

TOO MUCH STUFF

Dear Stuff,

Relax in your polar-fleece slacks, dude. Your roommate is just suffering from "I LOOOVE her" mania. It's very common. Someone finds another somebody and leaves behind a quivering little mass, writhing on the floor, yelping, "But I LOOOVE her/him."

The body's immune system then kicks in and all the red heartbroken blood cells get together and start pumping some type of disease-fighting distraction to the brain. For some, it's drinking. For others—like your roommate—it's shopping. (Oh, sorry, when a woman does it, it's called shopping. When a man does it, it's called buying stuff you really, really need.)

When the Nuisance Lady's old roommate, Sara, got dumped by her long-term boyfriend, she went to bed a somewhat normal girl and woke up a horrifying hybrid—part Martha Stewart and part Mother Teresa. She spent hours making splendid theme feasts: **Night in Bombay** (lots of stuff with curry), **Mexican Fiesta** (lots of stuff with guacamole), and Dim Sum Sunday (big disaster).

Then, after spending hours making little menu cards with sombreros and agonizing over squash versus pumpkin, she would invite homeless people off the street to join us for dinner. (Not that the Nuisance Lady's complaining, she met her last three boyfriends that way.)

This went on for six months until Sara met a new guy and ran out of recipes. Same thing'll happen to your roommate. He'll eventually run out of money, max out his credit cards, and meet a new chick. (Just make sure he pays his half of the rent on time.)

I'm with Her, Therefore I Don't Exist

Dear Nuisance Lady,

The other night I went out with my friend Lily. I met a really cute guy and we talked for forty-five minutes. At the end of our conversation he said, "So could I ask you . . ." Of course, I thought he was about to ask for my number. Who wouldn't? ". . . for your friend's phone number?" Can you believe that? And this is not the first time. Every time I go out with Lily, men surround her and ignore me. I don't get it. I really (I'm trying very hard to be objective) don't think Lily is that much more attractive than me. What's going on? I need to know because I'm starting to doubt my own attractiveness and hate Lily's guts.

THE FRIEND

■   ■   ■

Dear Friend,

Please, the Nuisance Lady was once trampled by an entire Australian rugby team madly dashing to her friend, terribly delicious Dana. Men have spilled drinks down the Nuisance Lady's dress in desperate attempts to get Dana's attention. One fellow even set one of the Nuisance Lady's eyebrows on fire with his cigar, frantically gesturing for the waiter to bring Dana another drink. And the Nuisance Lady's not alone; all of Dana's friends have similar stories.

And, believe it or not, Dana is not a knockout. She's sexy, but not overwhelmingly. She's pretty, but not too. She's smart, but not alarmingly. And that is the very secret of Dana's success—universal appeal. Some women just appeal to the male population at large. No doubt you are every bit as attractive as your friend Lily, but more specifically so. Maybe you have a caustic wit, a strong nose, a flat chest—something that does not necessarily appeal to Everyman. But even though only one man might be attracted to you for every ten that are attracted to Lily, that one is all you need; especially if he's a good one.

P.S. Bet you anything Lily—like Dana—has long, blond hair. Men love long, blond hair. They don't care if it's dyed, if the roots are down to there, if it's thin, or ratty, or on someone terribly tacky as long as it's long and blond.

Pale Blue Eye Shadow—I Looove It

Dear Nuisance Lady,

My friend Annie (I've changed her name so she won't kill me) does the worst makeup job you've ever seen. She wears bright orange foundation and smears it unevenly (very unevenly) all over her face. Then she lines her eyes with tons of bright blue eyeliner. Then she tops it off with glittery, goopy, bubble-gummy pink lipstick, which really, really clashes with the bright orange and bright blue she's got going on. Do you think I should tell her that her makeup is atrocious? I'm dying to. She'd be a pretty girl if she didn't make herself look like a carnival clown.

CAN'T MAKEUP MY MIND

Dear Makeup,

Never ever ever, ever, ever, ever, ever ever ever criticize another woman's hair, clothing, or makeup if you want to remain friends with her. Is that clear? These areas are just out-of-bounds. The Nuisance Lady learned this lesson the hard way. Once she tried to tell her dear friend Marcy from Great Neck that petite purple pedal pushers in a bold geometric print were not necessarily as flattering as one would like them to be. She smacked the Nuisance Lady over the head with her large leopardskin bag and screamed, *"This coming from someone who thinks cleavage is a verb."* It took months before the relationship was back to normal. Say something and you'll regret, regret, and regret again.

Let's Do Lunch—But Nothing Else

Dear Nuisance Lady,

I have a really good friend, Joe, whom I love hanging out with. We always have a great time together whatever we're doing—going to the movies, going for a few beers, etc. But lately I've been getting the feeling that Joe wants something more from our relationship. There are lots of signs, such as excessive criticism of all my dates, casual references to sex and stuff like that. I love Joe, but I just don't feel that way about him. Should I confront him or should I ignore it? If I ignore it and he makes a move, I'll die.

BUDDY-BUDDY

Dear Buddy-Buddy,

Remember the year when *When Harry Met Sally* came out and any and every reference to the movie would inevitably lead to one of your male friends trying to stick his tongue down your throat? Of course your friend Joe has a crush on you. This one-of-the-friends-wants-something-more thing has been happening ever since the early eighties. In the seventies everyone was so badly dressed, no one could find anyone else attractive; in the sixties everyone was so happy to be on the pill and be free that not having sex was not even a question; and before that there was no façade of platonic-ism, so men and women weren't even allowed to hang out together.

Don't address it unless he brings it up. If he does, just give him the old "I only want to keep on being friends" line. What else can you do? He'll either get over it or the friendship'll cool off for a while. It's all unavoidable.